Toys and Play for the Handicapped Child

BARBARA RIDDICK

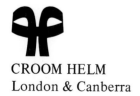
CROOM HELM
London & Canberra

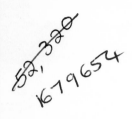

Croom Helm Ltd, 2-10 St John's Road, London SW11

British Library Cataloguing in Publication Data

Riddick, Barbara
    Toys and play for the handicapped child.—
    (Croom Helm special education series)
    1. Handicapped children — Education
    I. Title
    371.9   LC4015
    ISBN 0-7099-0292-1

Typesetting by
Elephant Productions, 93 Church Road, London SE19

Printed and bound in Great Britain
by Billing and Sons Limited
London and Worcester

Contents

Contents

Tables

Series Foreword

The Croom Helm Special Education Series is explicitly intended to give experienced practitioners in the helping services the opportunity to present a wide range of remedial programmes and techniques which they have developed in practice. The basis of the editorial policy is the belief that there exists much 'good practice' which warrants wider dissemination in book form so that its influence can extend beyond the local area where it is established. The present project is, therefore, concerned with the communication of ideas and methods developed by those who use them in their working lives.

Toys and Play for the Handicapped Child is written by a psychologist who ran the first professionally staffed Toy Library in the UK. Her experience enables her to write in practical detail about the role of toys and play, both in normal development and in the development of handicapped children. It will be found equally useful by parents, teachers and other professionals, and by those concerned to promote productive play in handicapped and non-handicapped children.

B.G.

Acknowledgements

This book has been written out of the experience gained in my work at the Nottingham University Toy Library and the Nottingham Melrose Centre for Handicapped Children. Therefore, the main debt is to the children and parents who have helped me to develop and refine my ideas on toys and play. Special thanks are due to Margaret Malkin and her son, James, who gave special help in the section on visual handicap; James appears on the cover of the book.

Mrs Wendy Foster and the staff of the Shepherd School, Nottingham, have been unfailingly helpful and co-operative. A general debt is due to the Child Development Research Unit, Nottingham University, and Beryl Bennett, Susan Gregory and Kay Mogford have been particularly generous in their help and advice.

Frances Croom typed a final draft from an ill-written manuscript; Sam Grainger took all the photographs in the book, a selection from many more: his skill and patience were much appreciated.

Finally, I am grateful to Bill Gillham who suggested I write this book in the first place and made sure I completed it. The final form owes much to the editorial skill of him and his wife, Judith.

B.R.

CHAPTER 1

Introduction

If we look at the normal five-year-old child he has clearly learnt an immense amount before he arrives at school. He can walk and talk, do simple drawings, play games, help dress himself and a host of other more detailed activities. How has he learnt to do all these things in such a relatively short space of time and, in most cases, without much formal instruction? Considering the large amount of time the pre-school child spends playing and rehearsing activities the answer seems, intuitively, that he must learn a lot of it through play. There is still considerable debate on how to define play and what its precise role is, but at a practical level it is certainly true that play is vital for a child's development and, to quote from John and Elizabeth Newson's well-known book *Play and Playthings*, 'play is perhaps the most serious and significant of all human activities'.

This statement appears paradoxical because the popular view of play leans towards the idea of it as something light and trivial. Perhaps part of the reason for this is that we take it for granted. We do not expect to have to 'teach' a child to play; it is something he does 'automatically'. By the same token we do not usually observe closely and analyse what is going on when a child is playing. Take, for example, the seemingly simple situation of a baby playing with a rattle. How did he get the rattle? Did he have it handed to him or did he pick it up from a surface? Did he reach and grasp for it accurately and easily or did he have to readjust his aim or did he fumble? What does he do when he is holding this rattle? Does he look at it fleetingly and drop it, or does he hold on to it and turn it round and seem to examine it closely from a number of angles? Does he mouth or suck it, or does he try shaking it to produce a sound, does he pass it from hand to hand, does he alternately glance at the rattle and at his mother as if to see her reaction? If he drops it does he look for it or, better still, look expectantly at the area it is likely to land in, or does he seem to forget it exists? These are but a few of the questions we can ask and which 'open up' the complexity.

To consider an example in more detail: if you give a young child three one-inch bricks, what is he likely to do with them? Some of the questions you could ask might be:

Were the bricks handed to him or were they placed on a surface for him to take?
If placed on a surface, how near or how far from him were they placed?

Were they presented one at a time or all three at once?
If all three at once, what did he do? Did he try to pick up more than one at a time in one hand or did he try to pick up a brick in both hands?
What did he do on picking the brick up? Did he examine it? Did he throw it? Did he pass it to his other hand?

The reason for asking all these questions is to work out what skills the baby has and what skills he needs to learn in order to do more things with the material.

(1) Whether the baby has learnt to co-ordinate his looking with his hand so he can grasp accurately.
SKILL: EYE–HAND CO-ORDINATION
(2) Whether the baby examines the object closely indicating that exploratory play is developing.
SKILL: EXPLORATORY PLAY
(3) Whether the baby looks for an object that has temporarily fallen out of his sight showing he has learnt that even when he cannot see an object it still exists.
CONCEPT: OBJECT PERMANENCE
(4) Whether the baby anticipates roughly where an object will land indicating that he is able to have expectations or make predictions about what is likely to happen in a given situation.
SKILL: PREDICTIVE SKILL
(5) Whether the baby alternately looks at his mother and the toy or object he is playing with indicating that he is learning to monitor social situations and is interested in the reactions of others.
SKILL: SOCIAL AWARENESS

Play and the Handicapped Child

The average child, given normal circumstances, seems to just get on and play without all this close observation and questioning being necessary. Children with handicaps, however, often have difficulty in playing and it is important that they should be given more structured help from an early age. Some may have difficulty in playing for mainly physical reasons. A cerebral palsied (spastic) child, for example, may have problems controlling his hands and a visually handicapped child because of his limited sight. Something that starts out as a physical disability can also affect a child's intellectual development because his chances to explore his environment and actively test out situations and try out ideas are limited.

Some children have physical problems which do not seem necessarily at first sight to affect play, but can in fact do so in less direct ways. The child with a heart problem or cystic fibrosis, for example, may be limited, especially during the winter, by the amount of time he can go out and the extent to which he can mix with other children so that his social play may suffer. Other children will have difficulties for mainly intellectual reasons so that although there is no physical reason why they should not play normally they seem to lack motivation or interest in playthings and find it difficult to work out what will happen or how they should proceed in an activity. These include children who are often referred to as developmentally delayed or mentally handicapped.

In a high percentage of handicapped children things are not as clear cut as this and they have some mental and physical impairment to varying degrees. This group would include those with Down's syndrome, some cerebral palsied children and some developmentally delayed children, some with spina bifida and many others.

But in all these children the important thing is to look carefully at what they *can do* and what they *can't do*. This probably sounds amazingly obvious, but learning to observe a child closely and to break down an activity into its component skills are the first steps, so that you can work out why a child cannot do something and what he needs to learn in order to do it. If, to take our earlier example, a baby does not reach for a rattle, we need to ask why. Is it perhaps because he cannot see it properly? Or is it because he cannot control his arm in order to reach for it? Or is it because he simply has no interest in reaching for it? Or is there some other reason?

Because play is such an integral part of a child's development, then, it should be taken seriously and not treated as something frivolous and irrelevant to the real business of learning. Many of the skills needed by the young in dressing, feeding and so on, are acquired through play. Learning to use his hands will start with the first rattle or the adult hand he plays with and proceed from there so that eventually he has the skills required to pull on a jumper, do up a zip, or fill a spoon and put it in his mouth. However, although play should be taken seriously, it should not be made into a serious activity: the essence of play is that it is something the child enjoys doing without pressure and constraint, something that is fun for him without necessarily having fixed goals. This balance has to be kept in mind.

Theoretically, toys as such are not necessary in order for a child to play. We all know how much young children enjoy playing with saucepans and the like, emptying cupboards and generally exploring household objects. In fact it is hard at times to draw a distinction between what is and what is not a plaything: Dad's motorbike helmet, the left over pile of building sand in the garden, Mum's rolling pin and pastry cutters, and so on. One sometimes suspects that toys were invented by adults to try and keep children away from valuable, breakable or dangerous objects. So, although various toys will be recommended as being useful for encouraging different activities, do not worry if you cannot obtain or afford them. Many other objects can be used as substitutes or other ways found of developing the same skills. It is also important to remember, particularly for the younger child, that toys are no substitute for an adult's attention. This sort of play does not have to be very formal and with most parents or caretakers is a natural part of their daily interaction with a child; for example, the common practice of 'playing aeroplanes' to get him to eat a spoonful of cereal. There is also a whole area of social play based on interaction with adults like peek-a-boo and pat-a-cake, and later interaction with older children.

Having worked in a Toy Library for the last five years, what has struck me forcibly is that although there are good and bad toys for a particular child, in many cases the way the toy is presented to the child by an adult and how he is helped to play with it is also very important. This does not detract from the fact that children do have strong preferences and that it is usually more productive to follow a child's particular interests (music, shape, colour) when giving him toys to play with. More discussion and information on choosing toys can be found in the final chapter.

How To Use This Book

If your child, or the child you are working with, is developing along roughly normal lines, albeit more slowly, turn to the age group most suited to him. The easiest way to find this out is to look at the outline of skills listed at the head of the chapters: the ages are, roughly, (i) babies, (ii) toddlers, (iii) pre-school and infant school age. For many handicapped children you may need to start at a younger age group than the one they are actually in, remembering that it is not a child's age that matters but what he can *do*, which is why it is suggested you check the list of skills involved for each age group. Again, you may well find that the child is relatively advanced in some areas and slower in others so you may need to consult two or more of the sections. If the child has a physical disability like cerebral palsy, visual handicap or deafness, as well as the appropriate normal child development sections, there is also a special section devoted to the specific difficulties and needs that arise from these types of handicap.

Areas of Play

Although a child may be learning several different skills whilst playing, it is useful to be able to break play down into specific skills or areas so that for any child his particular strengths and weaknesses can be pinpointed. The first major division that can be made, and the most important one to bear in mind, is between *social* (person) and *object* (toy) related play.

Children, especially younger ones, vary in the degree of interest they show in social play (i.e. play with other people) as opposed to play with toys and other objects. We all know the kind of child who plays for hours with his Lego or model farm as opposed to the child who seems to spend all her time rushing about with friends playing lots of imaginative games, and rarely sitting down for more than five minutes. For some handicapped children this difference is much more pronounced and is evident even in the young baby. Some show virtually no interest in toys and drop or throw most toys offered to them yet love adult attention and social games; others will be fascinated by certain toys and objects and play with them to the exclusion of everything else and will even reject or ignore adult attention or get annoyed if you try to play alongside them. These are obviously the extremes and most children fall somewhere between the two but it is useful to note whether a child has a strong leaning in either direction. Then, as well as building on the interests he already has, attempts can be made to involve him in activities in the areas he is missing out on (see also Chapter 2).

Besides this major division into social play and object-oriented play, play can also be broken down in a number of other ways. These divisions tend to be somewhat arbitrary and there can be a wide degree of overlap between areas but they can be useful as a rough way of labelling what the child is doing and giving the alert for areas he needs help in.

Exploratory Play

This sort of play is typified by older babies and toddlers who are attracted to all sorts of objects in their environment and actively explore them by picking them up and examining them. This examination can include mouthing and fingering toys, banging and rubbing on surfaces and throwing, often with interest in the results produced. Older children explore by crawling or toddling all over the house, opening cupboards and drawers and emptying out the contents, or exploring any new objects that have arrived in the home. In some children exploratory play seems to carry on predominating their repertoire longer than usual and they may need help in learning how to play constructively.

Constructive and Cognitive Play

It is sometimes hard to draw the line between exploratory and constructive play but, essentially, constructive play is more purposeful, as if the child has a definite plan or goal in mind or is working out how to formulate these. So, instead of just handling or pushing some nesting beakers round the floor he starts to try to put them inside each other or stack them all up. Fitting things together and learning the relationship between things will eventually lead to more complicated constructions like attempting to make things out of Lego, doing jigsaws or laying out a train set.

Social Play

Early examples of this are babies smiling in response to being tickled or spoken to in a special way. Later the baby learns to take an active part and will wave his hands or gurgle when it is his turn. Rough and tumble, hide and seek, etc. are later examples of social play. As well as social play with adults the pre-school child starts to engage in social play with other children, often in the form of imaginative or rule-following games. Children with older brothers or sisters are likely to be more 'sociable' in this respect than eldest or only children, because of their position in the family, but this is not always the case and individual personality is also a strong factor.

Imaginative Play

All sorts of imaginary games where the child pretends to be other people or pretends he is in a different environment come into this broad category. Early examples of imaginative play often seem to occur with toy cars, dolls or other models of people, and would include such things as pretending to go shopping, to give someone else a cup of tea or bandage up a toy animal who has 'hurt' himself. In the older pre-school child, games become more elaborate and often involve a group of children.

Gross Motor

Gross motor play includes such activities as running and jumping, climbing, riding a bicycle and dancing to music. It is a loose term to cover any large type of movements. The kind of skills required to indulge in this sort of play are good co-ordination and balance, and the confidence and interest to explore physical possibilities. Whereas some active children seem to spend all day engaged in gross motor play to the detriment of areas like constructive play, some unco-ordinated and apprehensive children will need a lot of encouragement in this area.

Language Play

In older children this is not strictly a particular area of play as language starts to mediate all forms of activity, but in younger children it is useful to delineate language as a particular area. Babies spend a lot of time babbling both for their own amusement and also as a social response to adults. They also derive great pleasure from imitating adult noises and having noises they produce imitated back to them.

Observing and Recording

At any given time a child might well indulge in an activity which involves several forms of play. For instance, he might start by exploring a toy and then go on to play with it constructively and as he does so he may also be talking to himself or may engage another person in the activity. This is why when presenting a child with a new toy or activity it is useful to be flexible in your expectations of how a child will play with it and what he will consequently learn from it. A marble run may seem at first sight very much a toy to encourage constructive play but in my experience it has often turned out to be an excellent toy for language play and social play ('your turn', 'my turn', 'stop', 'go', 'now', etc.). Conversely, it is useful to keep in mind those particular areas of play that you think need encouraging and either experiment until you find those activities that will do this or gradually work the play activity round to include those areas you want to develop.

Watch a child playing on three separate occasions for about five minutes each time, preferably when he is involved in different types of activities. See how many areas of play you can identify and label. This will help you to become adept at analysing play more informally while it is going on. Use the chart (Table 1.1) or draw up a larger one of your own to record and analyse in detail how a particular child plays. It will be more suitable for children over one year. Try to observe the child over the course of a day in a number of situations or, if this is not possible, for several shorter sessions. Pick a typical day: if the child you want to observe is very variable in performance try and record him separately on different days so that you can compare his performances. Tick and describe at least two incidences of each type of play. If certain types do not occur try to work out why. Sometimes it will be obvious, as for example with a physically handicapped child who is unable to walk, where gross motor and exploratory play are bound to be limited. But even in a case like this it is often possible to think of ways of encouraging these types of play to some extent. Various ball games could be tried for gross motor play and items like sand and water placed within his reach to encourage exploratory play. In the case of language and exploratory play, it may simply be that a child has not yet developed sufficiently. Sometimes the reasons for a child not engaging in certain types of play will not be obvious, although they can nearly

Table 1.1: Recording Types of Play

Type of Play	Tick two or more occurrences	Location	Time	What initiated it? (was it spontaneous or was it initiated by an adult or another child?)	Description	Any Difficulties
Exploratory						
Constructive						
Social						
Imaginative						
Gross Motor						
Language						
Any Other						

always be traced to a lack of motivation or lack of the necessary skills involved. When the reasons are apparent try to encourage the missing areas by placing the child in the best situation, making play interesting and demonstrating activities to him, giving the necessary help. The next chapter on teaching techniques will discuss ways of doing this.

Summary

Much of what a child learns is through informal play and playful exchange during daily activities like dressing, bathing and feeding. This extensive social play that goes on throughout the day forms an important part of a child's learning experience and should not be underrated or overlooked. Although less space has been devoted to this aspect of play, this is in no way intended to demean it but is a reflection of how much play is an integral and unself-conscious part of social interaction, and it is difficult, if not presumptuous, to lay down specific guidelines. Object or toy-oriented play, on the other hand, often has clear cut goals or sequences set by the material itself (e.g. operating a pop-up cone, posting shapes correctly). In these cases it is possible to look at what a child cannot do in terms of goals and sequences and the steps that can be taken to teach him.

The essence of 'teaching' a handicapped child to play is to keep a balance between structure and flexibility. Although you may have goals in mind, always be prepared to 'cash in' on any initiative or interest the child displays. Because play is engendered and fostered by inventiveness, enjoyment and surprise, an arid and rigid programme where goals are always set for the child may teach him specific skills but will not teach him how to play for himself in more informal settings. With slower children you may need to start by teaching specific skills but as soon as possible try to encourage them to use these skills in more informal settings for their own purposes.

CHAPTER 2

Teaching Techniques

More detailed and specific information on teaching techniques is given with each group of toys and play activities that are discussed, but to save constant repetition and to give general guidelines on how to approach teaching with a variety of toys and activities, this chapter is included.

Playing goes on all the time and shades into or overlays other activities like getting dressed or eating tea, but when thinking about how to help or encourage a child with his play it is probably easiest to start with straight-forward situations where you are specifically intending to play with him, and get used to applying certain underlying principles. When you find it comes fairly naturally these principles can be applied in a flexible and appropriate manner to other activities throughout the day.

Empathy and Communication

Perhaps the most important principle is to have *empathy* with the child — in other words, when you introduce a new toy or activity try to see it from his point of view. Does he really find it interesting or is it something you think he ought to find interesting? Are you pre-occupied with a goal you have set in your own mind (e.g. I want him to build a tower of beakers) or are you first watching to see what he does with the material and then picking up and follow-ing any initiative *he* takes? Sometimes mothers come back to the Toy Library and say a certain toy has been of no use. When we ask them exactly what happened we often find that the child did play with the toy in a variety of ways but not in the way they expected him to. He may, for example, have used some of the nesting beakers to make sand-pies or carry pebbles around in, instead of stacking them up as illustrated on the box; he may merely have put the pieces on and off the pop-up cone without attempting to fire it. Yet these other activities are valid in their own right: the toy has been useful in that the child has got something out of playing with it. Acknowledge, therefore, what he is trying to do with a toy by showing interest in it and approval and offering help where necessary, even when it is not quite what you expected.

Secondly, timing is very important. When you give a toy to a child watch carefully so that you can see when he will appreciate some help. It takes careful observation to avoid jumping in before he has really had a try at it, or leaving it until he gets frustrated and annoyed. The danger of jumping in too early is that you sometimes 'help' the child to do something completely different from what he had in mind. If a handicapped child is left to flounder for more than a few seconds, however, he may well lose interest in an activity without seeing its possibilities.

Communication will not be served by thrusting things persistently in front of a child's eyes or physically turning his head towards you. It involves making an approach and waiting for his reaction, or picking up any approach he makes to you, however slight. Keep the communication clear and at a level he will understand. If, for example, you want to point at the next piece for him to pick up, do not give a fleeting point while he is still looking at you. Make the point clear by waiting until he is looking at the piece in question. Similarly, with a child who is understanding only at a one- or two-word level, keep your requests simple. Instead of 'Now Mandy, are you going to be a clever girl and pick up the blue piece for me and put it in that box?' a simple request of 'Mandy, put the *blue* one in the box' or even, 'In the box, Mandy', pointing at the appropriate piece, would be better. Look out for the child's attempts to communicate as they may not be immediately obvious. He may look moment-arily at an out-of-reach object he is interested in or perhaps at you to indicate he wants something repeated. Alternatively, he might wriggle his finger or open his hand when he sees something he would like but not actually reach out for it. Again, the timing has to be right: telling a child the name of a toy when he has just glanced curiously at it will be a more effective communication than telling him when he is still engaged in some other activity.

Present things as clearly as possible from the child's point of view without causing him to become unnecessarily confused. Presenting three colour circles with three colour slots for them to go in may be an obvious colour matching task to an adult, but he may think you just want him to put the pieces back in and may not even notice or realise that *colour matching* is involved. You may need to hand him one piece at a time and physically guide him to put it in the correct slot; even this may have to be repeated several times before he notices that each piece is only put in the slot of the same colour. Help him as soon as possible to understand what it is you want him to do: with the three colour circles, for example, there is little point in letting a non-verbal child put all three in the wrong places and then telling him that he is wrong.

Make sure that the praise, encouragement and other rewards you give the child are noticed and interpreted as such by him. You may think that 'good boy' or a smile is praise and encouragement but he may not notice it or not perceive it as praise and may need something more attention-catching and forceful such as clapping or tickling. You can only decide what is rewarding to him by his response. Another child, for example, may find clapping and tickling overwhelming and will respond better to a quiet 'good boy' or smile. Most children tend to show which rewards they enjoy by laughing and smiling but some children do not do this and you can only tell by whether they carry on willingly with the activity you are rewarding or by more subtle signs such as hand-flexing or humming.

In summary, trying to see things from the child's point of view means incorporating some of the following in your approach:

(1) Making the activity interesting from the child's point of view.
(2) Being flexible as to the outcome.
(3) Following the child's leads.
(4) Helping when he *needs* help.
(5) Presenting things as clearly as possible.
(6) Reducing confusion for him.
(7) Acknowledging what he is trying to do.
(8) Giving praise, encouragement and other rewards that are seen as such by him.

Seeing the child's point of view does not mean doing what he wants all the time. It is a two-way negotiation and within reasonable limits he influences you and you influence him. You can work in quite a structured manner but, by allowing him to have some say in the proceedings, get better co-operation and results in the long run than if you directly demanded that the child do various things. Again this does not mean never asking or expecting the child to do something you want, but allowing him some leeway rather than getting into confrontation situations where any request may be met by defiance. Many parents and teachers are adept at employing diversionary tactics or making a game out of what they want the child to do or presenting it in an alternative manner. In the long run it is a much more productive approach.

Empathy is more important than having a lot of detailed knowledge about child development or a lot of special plans to follow. Many of the mothers who come to our Toy Library are excellent at teaching their handicapped children simply because they are already 'specialists' in their child and this enables them to work out for themselves the best way to help them. It might be, for instance, useful to know in a general way that babies first reach single-handedly to objects at the side of their body and at eye level and then learn later to reach objects placed in the middle at eye level and after this for objects at above and below eye level. An empathetic mother who does not know this may well work it out for herself: even though she may not realise it she will watch the child's attempts and automatically place the object at the best distance and angle for him.

A good example of a mother's natural ability to 'empathise' is shown in the accompanying illustrations. In the first photograph James and his mother look serious at the same time, whereas in the second one they are both laughing despite the fact that James is totally blind and therefore cannot see his mother's expression. In Photograph 1 James's mother was not certain what he wanted to do but she was watching him closely to pick up some clue. In Photograph 2 she had obviously found the right answer! Interestingly, an examination of about 40 pictures of James and his mother playing together showed they were either both smiling or both not smiling, which is an indication of how well-matched the mood of their play was. Without being consciously aware of it, it seems that empathetic mothers and adults continuously monitor their play interaction and constantly adjust it to keep it smooth running.

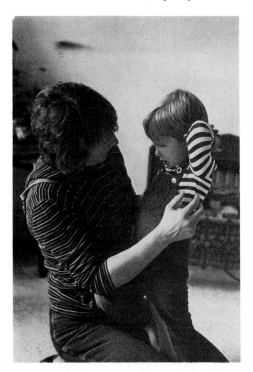 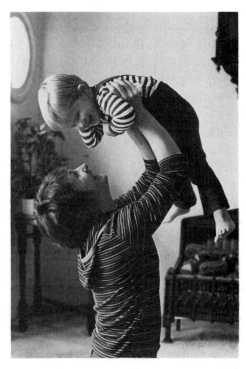

If you can tailor your interaction to fit in with the needs of a specific child then you can develop this skill even further. For example, if you know that the child deliberately engages or diverts you into an activity other than the one you would like him to do and you feel that he is missing out on certain skills, you could use a number of tactics to get him to do some of the things you think he would benefit from. We sometimes come across bright cerebral palsied children who, because they are very aware of their physical difficulties and have encountered failure in the past, constantly try to divert into conversation to avoid doing anything with their hands. By finding something enjoyable that is within their capabilities you can gradually build up confidence and skill so that this area is no longer something to be resisted. This is where it is important to think of games and toys that so absorb the child that he completely forgets about his difficulties. Children who have encountered failure are often anxious and wary, and resistant to anything they perceive as pressure to get them to do things associated with their area of failure.

Providing More Structured Help

We can now go on to consider the practical side of teaching techniques in more detail and think about how to adapt them to specific children.

To start with it might be useful to make a distinction between joining in and casually helping or showing a child what to do much as you would with any child, and sitting down with the express intention of teaching a child a particular skill. With some children all that may be needed is a little more help and encouragement than usual, whereas other children will obviously need more structured help. Children who hardly play at all, or who are easily distracted and inattentive, or are disorganised and destructive, or are severely physically handicapped, or flit from thing to thing, or are very obsessive in their play come into this second category. Much of what follows is common sense and applies mainly to these children who are going to need structured help in learning to play adequately.

(1) As mentioned before start by CLOSELY OBSERVING A CHILD. What can he do? What does he have problems doing? (Look at Table 1.1 and the Play Development Charts in Appendix B.)
(2) If he has NO OR LITTLE INTEREST IN TOYS OR PLAY you will have to gradually teach him.

For the child who likes playing with people but not with toys start by introducing toys that can be used as part of a social game such as rolling a ball backwards and forwards or pushing a car to each other. Encourage him to join in, not just watch the adult playing with the toy. Establish turn taking as part of the game. First you can make the cradle play spin round and then make it the child's turn. Later on you can develop more complex games, for example, encouraging the child to drop weebles down the weeble slide with you holding out your cupped hands or a tin to catch them. Similarly, you can play a game with the pop-up cone where you try and catch the pieces as they fly off. (In both these games the roles can be reversed.) The important thing for children like this is the adult involvement and interest in the toy and the whole social interaction surrounding it.

With children who seem largely to ignore toys, or are destructive, it is probably a good idea to reserve some of their toys for when you or another person have time to sit down and play with them with the child. It is usually better to keep back those toys the child finds more difficult and frustrating to use and let him have toys he knows how to use but is not yet bored with. Toys that 'do' quite a lot for a small effort on the child's part are often the best ones to leave the child to play with on his own, once you have taught him how to use them. The following toys are a few examples for each age group:

Babies

Activity Centre	Fisher-Price, Playskool and other makes
Chime Ball	Fisher-Price
Melody Push Chime	Fisher-Price
Maracas	Galt and others
Rattles	Various

Toddlers

Jack-in-the-box	Fisher-Price, Burbank and others
TV and Radio	Fisher-Price
Xylophone	Fisher-Price
Clic n' Clatter Car	Fisher-Price

Pre-school/Infant

Marble Run	Kiddicraft
Cash Till	Fisher-Price
Kermit Handpuppet	

Toys that require fitting and constructional skills and have various stages at which the child can get 'stuck' are often the least successful to leave the child alone with until he has fairly good mastery of them. Something like a pop-up cone tree, for example, can be very frustrating to a child if he cannot easily thread the pieces back on and, similarly, an inset or jigsaw that is too hard for the child to manage on his own can quickly lead to loss of interest or temper.

(3) If he is interested in playing with toys or objects but shows LITTLE INTEREST IN PEOPLE and generally resents being played with or helped, then toys will have to be used to build up social interaction.

With babies and toddlers you can start by capturing their attention by producing interesting effects with things they cannot yet work for themselves. Operating a spinning top, jack-in-the-box or musical toy are all good examples of this and with some babies, operating the various items on an activity centre can be a start. Basically, any effect that can be produced by a toy or object that is of interest to the child will do. Once he has shown interest, try to get him to communicate in some way if he wants a repeat performance. Do not push him or turn it into a confrontation situation but allow time for him to make a signal, however slight. To begin with it may just be a glance at you or the toy, the important thing being that you have started to build up a social interaction. Later try to encourage a point or a gesture or pushing of your hand towards the object and, with a speaking child, some relevant verbalisation (e.g. 'more', 'again').

Remember that most children like to play with toys on their own some of the time. When they are engrossed in what they are doing they may not welcome adult interference. With a few children, however, this is taken to extremes and they will refuse all help even when clearly 'stuck'. Screams ensue when anyone approaches, perhaps because they think the toy is going to be taken away. In these cases you can introduce a toy that a child can partly operate but needs some help with. A Jack-in-the-box where the child can let it jump out but cannot push it back in is a good example. Timing and patience are required: wait till he is stuck but try and intervene before he gets angry and annoyed or simply loses interest. Either do the bit he gets stuck on or, if he will tolerate it, help him to do it for himself. With some toys like a jigsaw or posting box, pointing to the correct slot or handing the child the correct piece in the correct orientation may be sufficient help. With other toys you may need to take the child's hand and show him how to do the activity. It is best to start with a quick straightforward activity such as just pressing a lever so the child gets the result he wants as quickly as possible. This is especially important with children who dislike being physically guided. Success does not always come easily and with some children merely turns into a battle, but if you can find a quick prompt and persist for several attempts the child may realise that you are not going to hinder him doing what he wants but actually going to help.

With a child who will not tolerate a physical prompt at all you can begin by presenting the material in the way that will make it easiest for him to succeed. In the illustrations John is being helped to thread size-graded rings on to a rocking post. He has a tendency to throw if he gets frustrated with what he is doing. Notice how his teacher is helping him by holding the rocking base still and lining the rings up in the correct order for him to put on.

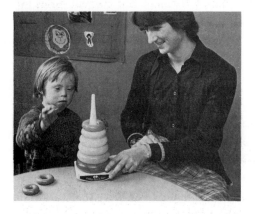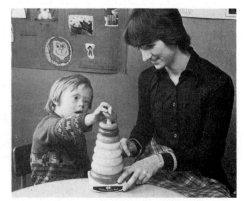

Breaking a Task Down into Easy Steps

This activity leads on naturally to the next area which is breaking an activity down into steps a child can manage. Quite often even when a child is initially interested in a toy he will rapidly end up throwing it and losing interest simply because he does not know how to play with it. If this happens often enough it tends to become an almost automatic response so if possible the adult should intervene before he has a chance to reject the toy.

Taking the seemingly simple task of John threading the rings on to the rocking post, it is soon apparent that a number of steps and skills are involved. John has to be able to use both hands at once, one to hold the base and the other to thread the rings. Prior to this he needs to realise that it is easier to thread the rings on if he holds the base still. He also needs to learn that the rings must be put on in descending size because the post is thicker at the base and the smaller rings will therefore get stuck near the top if put on first. One can imagine that left to his own devices John could have become frustrated very quickly when first given the toy. It is wise to allow a child some time to explore a new toy but this will vary from one individual to another. By grading the rings for him, and holding the base still, John's teacher has left him with the task of simply threading the rings on to the post. At first she might have made it simpler by giving him just a couple of the bigger and easier rings to thread on, or physically helping him to put them on. Later, she will probably teach him the steps of holding the base with his other hand and selecting the right size ring for himself.

This brings us back to the importance of observation. There is no point in helping or prompting a child with something he can already do but it is important to spot at what stage he gets stuck and why.

Take Eileen's teacher in these pictures, for example. First she lets Eileen, who is partially sighted, thoroughly explore this new toy on her own. Then she replaces the lid and watches her response. It is immediately obvious that Eileen will need to be helped to post the shapes through the correct holes so she takes Eileen's hand and physically guides her to do this before Eileen has had time to lose interest or get annoyed.

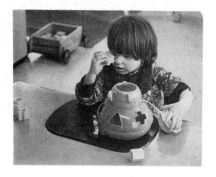 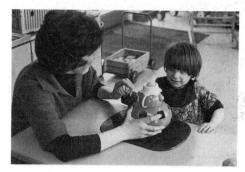

When a child is interested in a toy or activity but cannot manage it on his own, the first thing to do is always to ask how this can be broken down into easier steps or how you give the child additional guidance. Sometimes it may be the case that there are so many skills the child needs to learn that the toy is really beyond his present stage of progress. Again, by careful observation you will find that you become adept at picking toys that the child can eventually master, even when he needs initial help and guidance.

Motivation

The most important factor for success is your child's degree of interest. This can be *intrinsic* (inherent in the activity or toy itself) or *extrinsic* (dependent on praise, adult interest or small rewards). The ideal is for children to be self-motivated, i.e. interested in the activity itself, so they get intrinsic rewards from doing it. Having said this it is clear that many play activities are prolonged and given more excitement by an adult participating and showing positive interest and this is important if the child is to learn about all the subtleties of social interaction. Try a wide range of toys and activities to see what takes the child's interest. This is where the Toy Library can help if there is one in your area. Then, to increase motivation, present the toys and activities as interestingly and excitingly as possible; for example, letting the weebles rush down the weeble slide into a bowl of water is a lot more exciting that just plonking weebles and slide down in front of the child and leaving him to get on with it. Vary your presentation and the types of toy you choose: something that has little interest for the child on one occasion may be quite popular three months later when he has developed more.

Adult interest and praise are essential, though some children, especially those who seem to have no interest in social praise, are particularly hard to reward. With children like these you have to find things that are either rewarding in themselves or will serve as extrinsic rewards. Sometimes, ironically, it might be another toy. One boy I know works very well if allowed a short play with an activity centre between goes of learning a new skill. Another child may need to be rewarded by a short play of his favourite music, a sip of orange squash or a chocolate button. With all extrinsic rewards, give them as soon as the child does what you want him to do and at first give him a reward every time. Some children tire easily of one thing so you may need to alternate several rewards and make sure you only give a small piece of something to eat or a short-timed something to play with so the child is eager for more. Even if you have to help the child considerably by physically guiding his hand, still reward him every time or he will not learn that this is what you want him to do.

It is worth spending a lot of time and effort on finding ways of motivating the child because it will make it much easier for you to teach and encourage his play. Some handicapped children are notably difficult to motivate. I have come across bizarre rewards like flicking silver paper in front of their eyes, running their fingers through sand or watching a fluorescent light flicker on. The list is endless so there is plenty of scope for imagination. Do not forget that social interest and praise can take a wide variety of forms and, particularly with younger children, needs to be given very clearly and enthusiastically. With non-verbal children you need to use smiling, exclaiming, laughing, clapping, tickling and social games like round-and-round-the-garden, as well as verbal praise. In the illustration you can see how adult interest and excitement is being used to reward Claire.

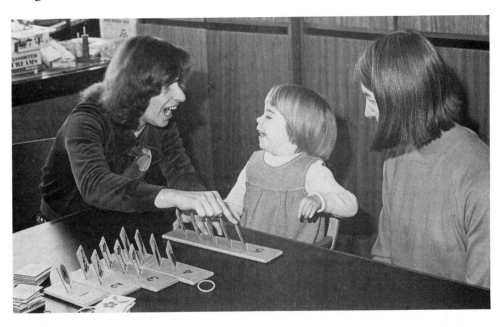

Presenting a Task

It has already been mentioned that the activity you want the child to do should be presented as clearly and simply as possible. If you look at the pictures of John with the ring stacker you can see that there is no other material on the table to distract him. This is especially important with a child who has poor attention and tends to flit from thing to thing. A table is not essential if you have a clear area of floor, but many of the mothers I have spoken to in the Toy Library do find that their child concentrates better if seated at the kitchen table or a coffee table or any other convenient surface in the house. One mother even used to work with her very active little boy in the bathroom as this was the least cluttered and distracting room in the house. Similarly, in nurseries, playgroups and schools, although an overall stimulating and interesting environment is aimed for, it is very useful to have a small room or sectioned-off area that is kept reasonably bare and distraction-free for individual work with children who have a poor concentration in their usual environment.

Both at school and at home, time of day is an important factor to consider. Particularly with hyperactive, lively children or unco-operative children it is useful to try and pinpoint a time when they are at their quietest or most co-operative. Some mothers and teachers claim that this is never! But these things are relative and, when pressed, most adults can name a time that is at least marginally better than others. This varies immensely: some mothers find that just after breakfast is a good time whereas others find just before bed is best. In nurseries and schools, teachers can often distinguish 'morning' or 'afternoon' children, or before or after break children.

Setting aside 10 to 20 minutes for individual structured play with a child can involve a lot of organisation and, at home, may not be possible if there are other young children to care for. Some mothers have found that when an older child is at playgroup or the younger baby asleep, they can set ten minutes aside for playing with the handicapped child on his own.

Having chosen a suitable activity you need to demonstrate clearly what you want him to do; with non-verbal children (children who do not understand language very well) you may have to use gesture or do the action several times to make yourself clear. It is important to make sure he is attending to your gesture or demonstration: this is where seating the child at a table can be helpful to focus the activity. If the task is one that involves several steps only give him the material that is relevant for the step he is doing to start with.

Prompting

Prompting includes any form of help or guidance you give a child. It can include physically guiding a child's hand to do something, pointing and gesturing or merely giving spoken guidance like a casual verbal prompt, 'Yes, on the green one' when you are encouraging a child to colour match. The degree and type of prompting will vary from child to child according to his own particular needs and difficulties. Prompting should not be used as a way of forcing a child to do something but as a way of helping a child to achieve something he wants to do.

Physical prompts (i.e. taking the child's hand and guiding it) can be used either to show a child what is required when demonstration, pointing and gesture do not seem to have made it clear, or to help a child who may know what is required but has not learnt yet how to physically make the response — as might be the case with a cerebral palsied child. Physical prompts can gradually be phased out until the child can do the activity by himself. A variety of prompts are often used even in teaching a child something quite simple. For example, if a child persistently tries to fit a piece of jigsaw in the wrong way round a verbal prompt may be given, 'Turn it round, Mary'. If there is still no response to this a turning motion may be made; if there is no response to this gestural prompt a physical prompt of helping the child to turn the piece round might be given.

Usually one starts by giving a verbal instruction or demonstration and then watches the child's response and quickly intervenes if the child needs more help. It is better to prompt generously when a child is learning a new task or activity and not let him flounder; later, when he has learnt the activity, you can gradually phase your prompts out.

Difficulties

'That's all very well but . . .'
'She throws everything she's given . . .'
'She never sits down for a minute . . .'
'She can break a toy in five minutes . . .'

Throwing and Destructiveness

Throwing can be quite a problem. The first thing to decide is whether this is an habitual, almost automatic, response or if the child only throws something when he is annoyed or wants attention. Try a period of ignoring it to start with. For this strategy to be effective it must be completely consistent in that the child is ignored on every occasion and preferably by everyone involved with him. Ignoring does not mean watching him out of the corner of your eye or sighing in exasperation each time he throws something. In fact it is best to look casually involved in an activity of your own as children are very quick to pick up the slightest signs of attention or annoyance. At first there may be an increase in the child's throwing as he waits for the response he normally gets, so again it is worth persisting for a month before you decide if this is having any effect. Occasionally, where throwing is not too much of a problem, parents and teachers find that a firm 'No' said before the child goes to throw can be effective. This is an alternative technique if you know it would be impossible for you to ignore throwing. Try either one method or the other consistently for a period, but not both together.

For both habitual and attention-seeking throwers another method is to present materials initially that cannot be thrown. You can do this with things that can be fastened down or that you can easily hold down yourself. A good example of the first is the Fisher-Price Activity Centre which can be fastened to a cot or chair, and of the second the Fisher-Price or Burbank Jack-in-the-boxes which you can hold down while the child operates them (see illustration). The advantage of both toys is that there are no spare pieces that can be thrown: unfortunately, there are not many toys that come into these categories so other methods are needed as well.

Many children seem to throw because they do not really know what to do with a toy or soon get bored with it. One way round this is to present the child with a new activity or toy only when you have time to sit down and teach him how to use it. Quite often if the base of a toy is held down and prompts are quickly given to the child to help him fit pieces in, throwing can be prevented. Sometimes throwing is a genuine indication of lack of interest, but it should be checked that the child has been shown the full potential of a toy as it seems that compulsive throwers do not give themselves a chance to properly explore a toy before throwing it.

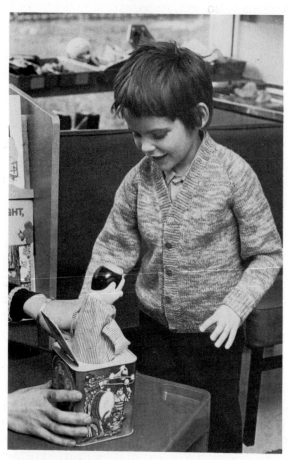

In the case of babies, throwing is, of course, a way of 'exploring' their environment, including toys. It is only when this throwing is so dominant that it prevents any other forms of exploration, or becomes dangerous, that it is a serious problem. One difficulty is that some children with slower cognitive development will require longer to explore their environment and will therefore be throwing objects when they are bigger and stronger than the average baby, and may also get stuck at this stage for quite some time. Down's syndrome children sometimes go on throwing long past the normal babyhood stage, probably because they need more help in learning how to play with toys.

Eliminating throwing can be a slow process and may in some cases take years of gradually teaching a child that there are more interesting things to do with a toy than throwing it.

Dealing with destructiveness towards toys has some features in common with dealing with throwing, in that you need to decide if the child is being destructive deliberately to get attention or is virtually unaware that he is being destructive. If his destructiveness is too frequent to be ignored, quietly remove the toy in question without paying him any attention and if necessary place the toy in another room. You may also need to remove any other toys or objects lying around if he is likely to transfer his destructiveness to them. Usually removing a toy for about ten minutes is sufficient time, though you may have to repeat the process before the child realises that the toy and your attention will be removed each time he is destructive. If attention-seeking is one of the main causes then give him a lot of attention when he is playing *constructively*.

With the child who hardly realises he is being destructive — what you might call an over-enthusiastic explorer of toys — a similar process can be used, but this time say 'No' clearly to him as you remove the toy. Eventually you may find that 'No' on its own will be sufficient and that you do not need to remove the toy as well.

Children Who Will Not Sit Still

Very active children are often referred to as 'hyperactive', although there is some debate as to precisely what this label means. Any parent who has a hyperactive child can certainly give a vivid description: and children like this do tend to rush from one thing to another, never giving themselves time to properly explore and play with individual toys.

With a child who has difficulty in concentrating, aim to keep him sitting for a few minutes only to start with; some parents find that a high chair right up to a table with a wall on one side and an adult on the other is a useful seating arrangement, making it more difficult for him to slip away. However, this should not be carried to the point of barricading him in as the idea is to get the child sitting because he wants to. Surprisingly, many hyperactive children once they have been seated and their interest engaged, concentrate quite well and perform much better than might be expected. The length of time the child will sit and concentrate for can gradually be increased and may then generalise to other more informal situations such as when he is playing with a toy on the floor.

Mouthing

Mouthing (i.e. taking objects to the mouth) is a normal response for babies and the average child does not stop mouthing completely until he is about

18 months old. With younger babies mouthing in the form of sucking and chewing seems to be related to comfort and to teething. Sucking as a form of comfort with specific objects such as a dummy or a piece of cloth or his own thumb may continue in some instances well past the age that a child stops mouthing other objects. For the young baby the desire to suck objects is a powerful one and it takes time for him to learn to inhibit this and start to explore toys purposefully with his hands instead. If follows that a baby who is developing more slowly than usual may well take longer to learn not to mouth nearly everything he picks up. For the child who has limited control of his hands and arms or shows little interest in toys, mouthing is at least a way of exploring toys and receiving stimulation, so one should be cautious about stopping it unless it is preventing him from exploring toys in other ways. For some physically handicapped children and blind children mouthing is a useful way of getting additional information about toys and objects.

If you want to encourage other forms of exploration, choose toys that cannot be taken to the mouth like the Fisher-Price activity centre, although some children are such keen mouthers that even with toys like this they will lean forward and suck various parts of it. Try to place the child in a position that makes this difficult to do, while still making it possible for him to explore the toy with his hands. Give him physical guidance and encouragement to do this if necessary. Play games with 'sound' toys like a tambourine where you take his hands and show him how to bang on it. Give him experience of different sensations using his hands, e.g. with water, sand, textured materials and so on, so that he gets used to and starts to enjoy exploring his environment in this way. Another task is to get him to *watch* attractive toys such as a perspex spinning top so that he becomes interested in looking at toys rather than putting them to his mouth.

Developing Your Own Techniques

Bearing in mind the practical advice given in this chapter and the principles of what we have called 'empathy', how then are you to begin developing your own teaching techniques? In selecting a new toy or activity appropriate to the child's level of development you can consider the following points:

(1) What time of day are you likely to pick?
(2) What sort of mood would the child have to be in?
(3) How would you get his attention?
(4) What sort of on-going activity is he likely to be engaged in? Would you wait for it to stop or would you interrupt it?
(5) If you needed to interrupt how would you do it?

(6) What location and setting would you choose? (E.g. alone together in the living room? In the bath with his brother?)

(7) Would you hand a toy to him or place it on the floor or table or somewhere else?

(8) Would you demonstrate how to use the toy first and if so how would you do this?

(9) If he showed no response to it, would you:

   (a) assume he had no interest in it and give up?

   (b) assume he had no interest but try to present it in a different way?

   (c) assume he had no interest because it was the wrong time or he was in the wrong mood and try it at some other time?

   (d) assume he did not know what to do with it and show him by prompting?

(10) If he started to play with it but not very competently what would you do?

(11) If he started to play with it quite adequately what would you do?

These are but a few questions that can be asked and show how much thought and observation needs to go into helping a child play. Most of the time we do this unconsciously but with children who need more help than usual it is particularly important to be aware of how much is involved in seemingly simple activities. This may seem a bit odd at first but soon becomes quite automatic and blends into one's normal interaction with a child.

These notes are merely to give some guidelines, of course, and are not intended as a rigid set of rules which must be followed. Children vary so much in personality and interests that what works well with one child may be a disaster with another. Many nurses and teachers have developed their own individual ways of helping young handicapped children to learn to play, which are based on their own characters and abilities and are tailor-made to suit the needs of different children. Some children respond better to parents as teachers, and indeed parents have some advantages over professionals particularly where children have special difficulty in expressing their needs; however, if attempts at structured teaching at home lead to confrontation and upset it is probably wise to stop. As with many normal children who refuse parental help with reading and writing, some handicapped children do not respond well to structured teaching by their parents.

CHAPTER 3

Babies (0-12 Months)

Skills to Develop

(1) Watching and following objects and people with his eyes.
(2) Head control, arm and finger control, rolling and sitting up.
(3) Grasping, mouthing and exploring objects.
(4) Simple social responsiveness, smiling in response to adult greeting, etc.
(5) Listening to the sounds things make.
(6) Shaking or banging an object deliberately to produce a sound; a rattle for example.
(7) Babbling and making noises in response to specific events.

These are just some of the most basic skills that develop during the first year. If the child you are going to work with already has all these skills, check the list at the beginning of the next chapter on *Toddlers* and move on if appropriate.

Starting Off

Clearly the baby needs to be in a comfortable and well-supported position if you want to encourage play. It is particularly important to do this with a 'floppy' baby who may be late in sitting up. Most mothers are good at finding what position their child prefers to be in and improvising to give sufficient support. Sometimes wedging a baby in the corner of a settee with additional cushions for support is fairly successful. If he is still not sitting unsupported well past the average age (6-8 months) and is still very 'floppy', the health visitor or GP can be consulted: they may refer on to a physiotherapist for advice. For some children who have particular difficulty in sitting, special types of seating are available and physiotherapists usually know about these.

Anticipation Games and Social Play

Social play with an adult is the first and most important type of play a baby is involved in. Particularly during the first few months, he will have little interest in objects but will be fascinated by people. Whereas he has not learnt how to control objects, he finds that people will respond to his gaze or movements, predictably but with enough variation to keep him interested and often excited. Early smiling, face pulling and tickling games can lead on to anticipation games where you creep your fingers up the child's leg and then tickle his tummy or circle your finger towards him and touch his nose; these are great favourites and often have him laughing long before the final touch. A sense of timing about how quickly to build the game up to its climax and how quickly to repeat it soon develops between a mother and her baby.

Another surprise game most babies love is peek-a-boo and endless variations on this can be played. Later copying lip-smacking and other sounds the baby makes will also be enjoyed, as will turn-taking games where he hands you an object and you then hand it back. It is easy to make this more exciting and keep the game going longer by, for example, hiding the preferred object behind your back for a moment and then producing it with a big exclamation of surprise.

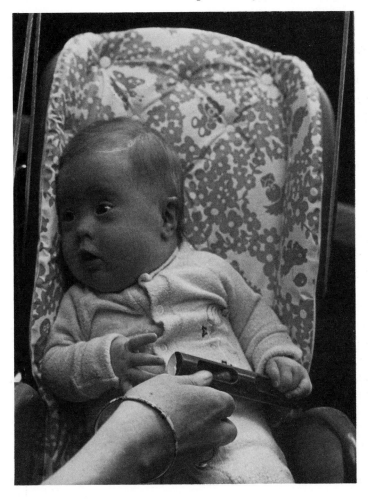

Handicapped babies need the same sort of social play as other babies and some seem to respond well to it compared with their rather slow start with object play. In the illustration Richard is clearly more interested in the adult handing him the rattle than in the rattle itself! Other handicapped babies are rather passive and may not seek out and initiate social play in the way that the average baby does, so you may need to 'take the play to them'. You may also need to be alert to very faint signs that he is enjoying a sequence of play, such as a fleeting smile or a slight turning of the body towards you. Some handicapped babies respond well to quite rough play like being thrown in the air or jiggled up and down. As with any other baby it is necessary to be sensitive to his reactions and not to force games on him that he does not enjoy. Because some babies are slower to learn it takes them longer to understand facial expressions and movements and things need to be louder and clearer to catch and hold their attention. This means that social play may need to be slightly exaggerated with clearer signals to get the baby's attention and loud exclamations to mark what is happening. Sequences of activities will need to be built up more gradually and carried out more slowly so that the baby can follow and enjoy them. All babies like to have some control over the social play situation so care must be taken not to 'impose' play on them that they are reluctant to join in with. There is a thin line between stimulating or encouraging play and 'imposing' it: it is a matter of picking up the signals the baby makes, however slight, and responding to them sensitively.

A small number of babies seem to have an intense dislike of being picked up. They squirm and arch their back and sometimes cry until put back in their cot. In this case one can play social games when the baby is in a cot, on the floor, lying on a 'sag-bag' or in a baby relaxer chair — wherever, in fact, he seem happiest.

First Toys (Mobiles, Mirrors, etc.)

Babies spend a lot of time looking around them at the environment and what is happening. Research has shown that even very young babies prefer to look at patterned as opposed to plain things, so from early on you can hang up mobiles or anything else that is bright and colourful and catches the baby's attention.

Make sure the mobile or mirror is positioned so it is in the baby's line of vision and does not require him to turn his head or body awkwardly. It is a good idea to change regularly the sort of things you have hanging up as the baby will probably get bored if it is the same thing all the time. You could improvise with a ball of silver paper on a string or some bright squares of cardboard cut from cereal packets, or even an interesting rattle or colourful small toy. Some children take less interest than others and it may be necessary to try a whole variety of objects before you find anything they are interested in.

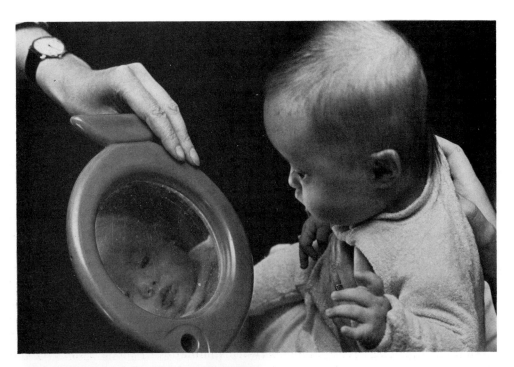

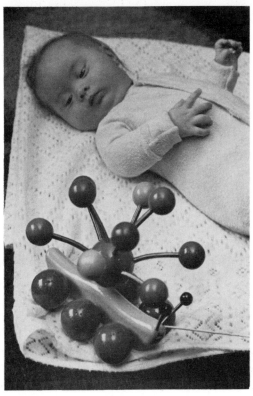

See if the baby is able to follow the mobile, object or toy when it is moving. This is called *visual tracking*. Does he follow it if it moves from side to side? This *horizontal* tracking is usually the earliest type of tracking movement a child can perform. After this comes *vertical* tracking — following an object up and down with his eyes.

To start with make sure the child is looking at the stationary object and then move it slowly in front of his eyes. Try it about a foot away from his face but move it closer or further away if he seems to follow it better at a closer or greater distance. Some children seem better able to track to one side than the other. If this is the case, encourage the baby to track in the direction he does not normally follow. Once he is following moving objects from side to side and up and down see if he can track them if they move in a circle. You will probably need to hold an interesting toy or object in your hand in order to do this although you can also do it with things on a short piece of string. Finally, see if the child can follow things if you zigzag them about in no predictable pattern or direction. If the child has difficulty with tracking and needs practice at it make more of a game and accompany presentation of objects with smiles, exclamations and noises to hold his interest.

Visual tracking is one of the earliest skills a baby will learn and before he starts to track objects you will probably find he is 'tracking' or following you or other familiar adults with his eyes. Where possible lay or prop him in positions where he can do this.

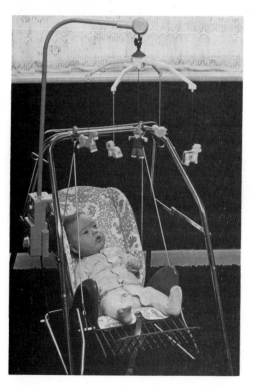

Mothercare sell a cot mobile (£2) and also a musical cot mobile (£3.85). Kiddicraft also produce mobiles and a lot of gift and craft shops sell mobiles. Fisher-Price manufacture a musical mobile that can be attached to a cot or any other convenient surface (see illustration). It is rather expensive but would be useful for a child who particularly enjoys music and needs extra encouragement at tracking as the pieces revolve slowly.
Skill taught: VISUAL TRACKING

Cradleplays

Cradleplays have some of the properties of mobiles in that even before a child is ready to reach out and play, he can look at the cradleplay and also watch as an adult sets certain parts of it in motion. Apart from the fact that they can all be fixed across a cot or pram, cradleplays come in a wide variety of shapes and sizes with differing activities on them, although most involve some sort of spinning or revolving activity and some sort of noise-producing activity. They are an invaluable first toy for two reasons: the child has only to make a fairly rough swipe at it in order to produce an effect and, because they are firmly attached in place, they do not roll or fall out of the child's reach.

A normally developing baby woud probably start to use a cradleplay at about 6-9 months. If a handicapped baby does not start to play spontaneously with the cradleplay after a few demonstrations it is worth reviewing why this might be. For instance:

Does he seem to show no interest in it at all?
Does he try but is unable to hit it and produce an effect?
Other reasons? E.g. has he grown so used to it that he has lost interest?

The first two reasons are common in slow developing children and underline the point made in the introduction that some children need to be *taught to play*. Obviously this is a question of degree as even an advanced baby will sometimes need a little help, but the more difficulties a child has the more help he may need.

First check the positioning of the baby and the cradleplay to make sure that his lack of interest is not simply because he cannot see it properly. It is useful to have two adults engaged in first presenting a cradleplay, one with the baby seated comfortably on their lap facing the other adult who holds the cradleplay out to the child. This way it is easy to adjust the distance of the cradleplay from the child and direct his attention by moving the various parts yourself and exclaiming and smiling as you do so. This will be particularly important if he is the sort of child who displays little interest in objects but a lot in people. In other words, use *your* interest in the toy to try and focus the child's attention and interest on it.

If the baby makes unsuccessful swipes at the cradleplay try to position it so it will be in the arc of his movement and praise him if he hits it. If he is very inaccurate or makes no attempt to play with it but *looks* at it with interest, gently guide his arm or hand to set something in motion. Do not try to force the baby to do it if he resists or shows no interest at all. You may need to guide his hand several times before he will start attempting to swipe at it for himself. If he tries but misses through inaccuracy try gently guiding his arm by holding it at the elbow.

Skill taught: EYE–HAND CO-ORDINATION

Rattles

There is a bewildering variety of rattles on the market. The rattles illustrated are some of the ones we have found most useful in the Toy Library, although plenty of other equally useful rattles exist. Generally speaking, those produced by well-known manufacturers such as Kiddicraft, Mothercare, Playskool, ESA, Fisher-Price, etc. will all have been carefully tested for safety. With little-known or unnamed makes, check that the rattle is not made of thin brittle plastic which will splinter easily, or coated in toxic paint or fitted with small pieces which might easily become detached and swallowed.

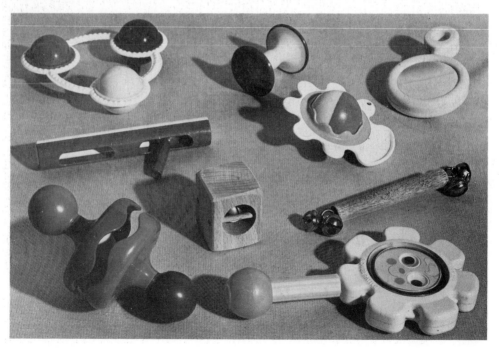

Choosing rattles for a particular child tends to be a somewhat hit-and-miss affair. Some babies seem to like almost all rattles handed to them whereas others are very selective and have a few or even just one favourite. The average baby can usually play happily with a rattle by six months. As a rule, with a younger baby or a child who seems reluctant to handle a rattle it is better to choose a very light one. The three ball rattle is an example of a very light rattle which produces a lot of sound from even slight shaking. It also has some thin parts on it which are easy for the child to grip. The small dumbell rattle and mirror rattle are also fairly light and easy to produce sound from.

The clic-clac rattle and the Japanese wooden rattle both have interesting sounds but require slightly more purposeful shaking in order to produce them. They are fascinating rattles for a baby to watch and provide new stimulation and feedback for a baby who has mastered the simpler rattles. Another set of rattles which often interests babies are those that have something visible inside an outer casing. The square bell rattle and the ball in a circle rattle are examples of these and so is the clic-clac rattle mentioned before. Some larger rattles like the swirl rattle are useful for encouraging two-handed play. A number of rattles like the flower rattle and the ring-a-ling rattle are also designed as teethers. A very light maraca also makes a good rattle.

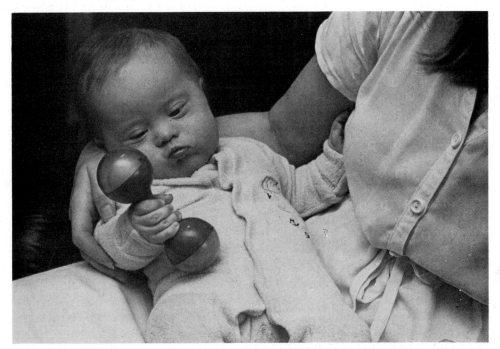

Some children will need no help — just hand them the rattle and they will do the rest! But if your child is not playing with rattles first try and decide why. Is it because he has no interest in rattles? Or is it the case that he is interested but lacks the skills necessary to enjoy them? Try out a wide variety of rattles. Some babies are primarily interested in rattles as visual objects (something to look at) whereas others are more interested in the sounds they produce. Shake the rattle yourself at different distances and positions from the child. Play games where you suddenly produce it from behind your back. Anything in fact that will get his attention. You may have to put the rattle in the baby's hand and help him shake it and repeat this several times before he will become interested and realise that he can produce interesting effects by shaking it himself.

Some children dislike new and unfamiliar things and will tend to reject any new toy out of hand. Leave the toy lying around for a few weeks, then play with it yourself in front of the child and see if he starts to show interest in it. If he does you can then encourage him to play with it. With some children you may need to introduce the rattle several times before they will accept it.

If your child has difficulty in reaching and grasping for a rattle you can try different shaped rattles to see which one is easiest for him to hold. There are a number of suction rattles on the market which can be attached to most smooth surfaces if the child is having real difficulty in holding on to a conventional rattle. In fact one of these is useful for most babies as their favourite game of dropping toys or casting them away means that if no willing adult is available they soon have nothing to play with. However, do not *discourage* the child from playing dropping games once he is capable of playing with a rattle: he learns a lot from this and from about ten months onwards realises that an object that falls from sight still exists (object permanence). He is also learning about cause and effect, i.e. 'If I drop this rattle on to the floor it will produce such and such a noise'. It is also a good way of learning an early turn-taking game with adults: 'If I drop this rattle she will pick it up and hand it back to me'.

Skills taught: EYE–HAND CO-ORDINATION
OBJECT PERMANENCE
CAUSE AND EFFECT
EARLY TURN-TAKING GAMES

Dangling Toys

Dangling toys fall into two main groups: those that are specifically designed as dangling toys, such as the Fisher-Price Jumping-Jack Scarecrow and Pull-a-tune Bluebird or the Kiddicraft Swing-and-play; and a whole variety of small toys and objects which although not designed specifically for this purpose can easily be suspended by a piece of elastic or string. Since they are the most readily available we will consider the latter group first.

Anything that can be suspended and takes the child's interest can be included in this group. Small toys like rattles and squeakies are an obvious choice but many items available in the house such as rolled up balls of silver foil, old smartie tubes and so on can be used. Where and how you suspend the toys will depend on the skills and mobility of your child. One mother I know hangs a number of things on a baby bouncer frame and lays her handicapped son on a small mattress in the middle of it. Another mother suspends a sort of low level washing line across part of her living room with articles dangling from it; this is particularly useful for the more mobile child whose mobility needs encouraging. You may need to make a small frame to suspend the toys from for a cot, pram or chair. Make sure in this case that the objects are near enough to be easily seen and grasped. In the illustration Brian is playing with a suspended plastic bottle which is filled with colourful beads.

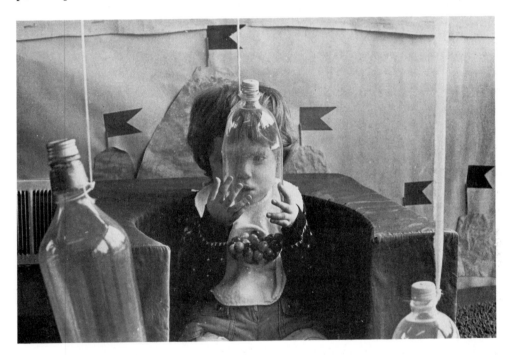

There are quite a few 'purpose-built' dangling toys available now so only those that we have found particularly successful in the Toy Library are mentioned here. One of the largest groups of dangling toys are of the music box variety where the child pulls a string so that it plays a tune. One problem with many of these is that the string with its attendant knobs or handle is far too stiff for the child to pull, so try it out first yourself with a very light tug, before buying. A good example of one of these music box toys is the Pull-a-tune Bluebird (Fisher-Price). This has a large brightly coloured handle which is fairly easy for the child to grasp and does not require too hard a pull to set it going.

Other dangling toys also produce a visual effect, like the Jumping-Jack Scarecrow (Fisher-Price), whose arms and legs shoot up in the air when the string is pulled. Raymond, a cerebrally palsied boy, is shown playing with one of these with obvious enjoyment, after his teacher had guided him by holding the handle steady and helping him to give it a downward pull. Inaccurate grabs will, of course, set the handle swinging making it even harder for the child to grasp — hence the importance of a vigilant adult. Raymond's handicap, in this respect, puts him on a par with much younger children, but the principle remains the same.

Skill taught: EYE–HAND CO-ORDINATION

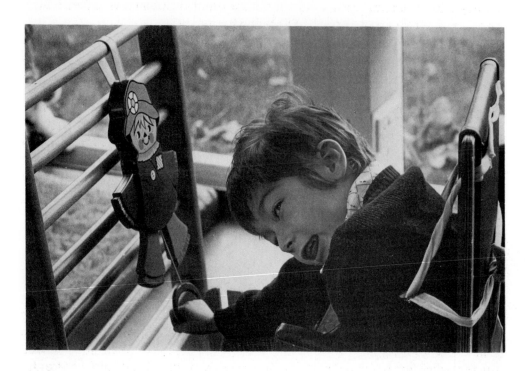

Following On

As the child learns to control his responses to the first toys that are presented to him, so he will become capable of enjoying playthings that demand a more complex response. The second half of this chapter makes suggestions of toys to follow on with.

Activity Centres

These are a relatively new type of toy although enterprising parents have long constructed their own for babies and handicapped children. Activity centres although reasonably expensive (about £6–£10) are often a good investment for a number of reasons. There are several different activities of varying degrees of difficulty on the centre so they provide a wider range of experiences on one toy. Most are attachable in some way to a cot or chair and even when free will not roll out of the child's range so that they are particularly useful for the non-mobile child. The better makes such as Fisher-Price and Playskool are very durable and rarely break. One of the earliest was the fix-on one by Fisher-Price: this is still widely available and one of the best in terms of value for money and durability. Fisher-Price have just brought out another called a Turn and Learn Activity Centre which rotates on its own base.

Because you cannot actually 'hand' an activity centre to many younger children, placing them in exactly the right position is very important. If you have a very floppy baby or child who is not easy to support you may find that at first you will need to hold the centre in the best position for them. Most activity centres have one or two items that just require an easy swipe to set them going, then several more difficult items that require pulling, pushing, twisting, etc. which may take much longer to master. One advantage of an activity centre is that for many children it is not a toy that requires a lot of teaching on how to use it and is best left within their reach until they show spontaneous interest in it.

Skills taught: EYE–HAND CO-ORDINATION
CONTROLLED MANIPULATION

Balls and Roly-Poly

A light brightly patterned football-size ball makes an excellent toy and needs no introduction. There are also a variety of noise-producing balls such as the Chime Ball by Fisher-Price. This is a heavily weighted ball that is not intended for throwing but is for babies to push or rock with their hands or feet in order to produce a sound, and also to watch the small figures inside (e.g. a rocking horse) move.

Many of the roly-poly toys work on the same principle as the Chime Ball. They have a heavily weighted base and are often in the shape of something like a bear or duck. The toys are for pushing or rocking and the figure leans right over when pushed but eventually comes back to rest in a vertical position. The Chime Ball, the Roly-poly Chime toy and the Happy Apple are also watertight and can float in the bath. These sort of roly-poly toys are useful for children with restricted mobility because they do not roll out of reach, and are useful for children with poorly co-ordinated movements because a swipe is all that is needed to set them in motion. You can also use the roly-poly for simple copying and turn-taking games. You can knock it over and then wait to see if the baby will do likewise; if he does you can then praise and exclaim and knock it over in turn again. If not, repeat the process several times. If he is not interested and excited, take his arm and show him how to hit it himself.

Another interesting kind of ball not intended for throwing is the Baby Action Ball. This has outer plastic slats that make it easy for the child to hold, and an inner perspex area shaped like an egg timer though which small plastic chips filter if the ball is tipped up. This is visually interesting for children and many like the rustling sort of sound produced as the chips pour from one end to the other. The only disadvantage is that for younger children it can be rather heavy and you may have to start by holding the ball yourself. Another ball that is similar in shape to this is called a musical ball and produces sounds when shaken or rolled.

Children also like the Discovery Ball which is made up of several plastic pieces and a central rod which can in fact be used on its own as a very effective rattle or will produce sound as an integral part of the ball. There are also a number of balls like the one produced by Mothercare which have ridges just the right size for a child to grip. Most of these will make a sound when squeezed.

If the child you are dealing with cannot hold anything heavy a very light foam plastic ball which is easy to grip may be a useful start or, alternatively, a light washable material ball. These often have a bell inside as well. Another idea is one of the small hollow plastic balls which have a number of holes on the surface.

Table 3.1: First Balls

Toy	Manufacturers	Suppliers or Shop
Roly-poly	Various	General
Roly-poly Chime	Mothercare	Mothercare catalogue or shops (£1.95)
Happy Apple	Fisher-Price	Various shops
Easy grip type ball	Various (including Mothercare)	Various shops, Mothercare, ESA catalogue
Chime Ball	Fisher-Price	Various shops
Musical Ball	Various	Various shops, ESA catalogue (£1.55)
Baby Action Ball	Playskool	Various shops, ESA catalogue (£4.77)
Material balls	Various	Various shops, ESA catalogue, Mothercare catalogue (set of four £5; hanging ball £1.45)
Perforated plastic balls	Various	Various shops, Galt catalogue ('gamester ball' 86p per set)
Discovery Ball	Four to Eight	Four to Eight catalogue

With most of the specialised balls it is simply a matter of introducing them to the baby and seeing if they interest him. An ordinary light plastic ball, preferably brightly patterned, is ideal for establishing early ball rolling games which will encourage turn taking and anticipation. Although these are possible from a prone position the best position is with the child sitting on the floor with his legs apart. You can then roll the ball gently to him so that it is caught by the V formed by his legs and will stop right in front of him. At first draw his attention to the ball when you are holding it and say something like 'ready' when you are going to roll it. If his attention is very fleeting you may need to tap the ball on the ground to get his attention when you are going to roll it. Encourage him to follow the ball with his eyes from when you release it until it arrives in front of him. Some young children find it very hard to switch their attention and will still be staring steadfastly at you as the ball rolls towards them. Draw their attention back to it by looking at the ball yourself and pointing and exclaiming. Even when the child watches the ball quite carefully it is often some time before he learns to co-ordinate his hand movements with his gaze; in many cases it will be his body that stops the ball and he will then reach down to it with his hands.

Sit quite close to the child and encourage him to roll it back by holding your arms out and urging him to do so. If this gets little response you may need to help him yourself. Ideally the game is better if two adults are present, one to sit behind him and show him how to push or roll the ball while the other is in front ready to catch it. This is also a good plan if you have a floppy child who is slow to sit unsupported. How the child actually propels the ball tends to vary. Some start with a backward swipe of the hand whereas others push with either one or both palms. If you need to physically prompt the child do whatever seems to suit his natural arm movements best. If in doubt a backward swipe is probably easiest for a child with poor arm control, although later try to encourage proper rolling. By sitting near him you should with a bit of alertness (and a few dives!) be able to catch most of his attempted rolls as at first he will have little control over their direction.

This activity is a good way for the child to learn a turn-taking type of interaction. A child who does not respond in this situation may be one who is slow in picking up social signals — being aware of what other people want — and this is a useful way to begin teaching him these sorts of skills.

Skills taught: EYE–HAND CO-ORDINATION
               TURN TAKING
               ANTICIPATION
               VISUAL TRACKING

Early Push and Pull Toys

Although push and pull toys are more appropriate for toddlers (see p. 73), some are included here because they can be used by a baby or non-mobile child simply as a static toy and are also useful for encouraging crawling.

Some of the best pull-alongs are produced by a Greek firm called Kouvalias. They tend to be stocked by bigger toy shops and department stores. Many of the Kouvalias toys are characterised by brightly coloured wooden balls and the like on strong springs attached to some sort of wheeled base that can be pulled along. The illustration shows Eileen exploring the pull-along Cricket for the first time. The advantages of a toy like this are that its bright glossy colours make it attractive to many children and that a mere swipe of the hand or arm will set the balls in motion so that they bob about on the springs and make a clacking noise as they hit each other. Later, when the toy is pulled along, the balls rotate on their base. So far no one we know has managed to remove any of the balls from the springs so they must be quite strongly attached and the paint is non-toxic.

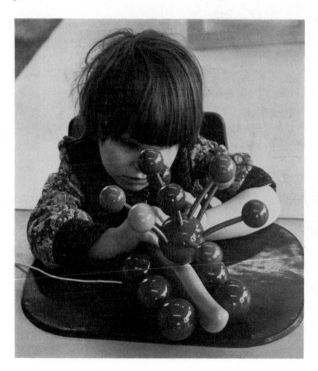

There are various Kouvalias pull-alongs: one has rotating mushrooms on springs which hit a ball; another has rotating balls in the shape of a windmill that hit a bell as they turn round. Another very attractive pull-along is the Kiddicraft 'Clatter Pillar'. This also has two small balls on springs for antennae and these are very attractive to children but beware if your child is particularly strong. When the toy is pulled along it wobbles from side to side and makes a clattering noise. Here it is being used to encourage Eileen to crawl. Later this toy is popular with toddlers as a conventional pull-along.

The point about all the pull-alongs mentioned so far is that they are sufficiently interesting to take the child's attention even before he is old enough to pull them along. There is a wide variety on the market. Brio, for example, produce some attractive ones so shop around and see what you can find. The Kouvalias cricket, at around £8, is rather expensive; however, if you have a child who is particularly hard to interest in toys or has such poor control over his arms and hands that he cannot play with them very effectively, then such a toy might be a good buy and will certainly last well.

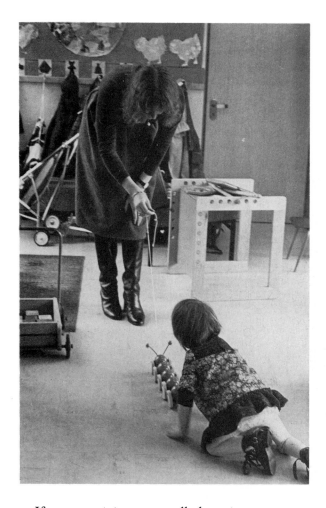

If you want to use a pull-along to encourage crawling or some other way of moving around the floor, choose one the child is obviously interested in and has had time to explore but is not yet getting tired of. Do not use this as a method on a child who has shown no sign of moving in the desired manner before: it is best used with a child who has just started to crawl but only does it very occasionally when sufficiently motivated. At first only induce the child to crawl a few feet and then let him have the toy as a reward for his effort. If you keep it at a fun level he will often be quite happy to repeat the exercise several times and with extended lengths of crawling. The important thing is to monitor carefully the child's response and not let him reach the point where he is angry and frustrated at not getting the toy.

Fisher-Price have recently brought out a new toy called a Bob-along Bear which is a cross between a pull-along and a roly-poly. The slightest push back or pull forwards will cause the arms to rotate, and a baby by merely swiping it can set the bear and the balls in the perspex hemisphere in motion. It is a good pull-along to start teaching a child to pull by the string from a sitting position.

You can place the bear about six inches to a foot outside the child's reach, then put the string into his hand as near to the bear as possible and show him how to pull it towards himself. After the first demonstration, when you place his hand on the string again pause and see if he will pull it for himself before helping him. You can encourage the child to sit with his legs splayed so he pulls the bear in front of him or with legs together so he can pull the bear to the side of him if this seems more comfortable. Either way you will probably have to put the bear back ready for another pull. If he is enjoying the game you can then encourage him to push the bear back for another turn, and finally see if you can get him to pick up the string for himself. The string on most pull-alongs is usually too long for a child who is pulling from a sitting position so shorten it if necessary and tie a large wooden threading bead or something similar to the end to make it easier to grasp. On the Bob-along Bear, for example, you can double the string up and tie a knot at either end to hold both strands together. Do not be discouraged if at first the child spends hours playing with the string and nothing else as babies love playing with string and presumably learn quite a lot from the experience.

Skills taught: MANIPULATIVE SKILLS
THE CONTROL OF LARGE MOVEMENTS
(e.g. ROLLING OVER, CRAWLING)

Music Making Toys

It is hard to decide where rattles and the like stop and music making toys begin. It does not matter much for the purpose of this book, and quite a few useful toys for babies are to be found under the heading of music making toys. Galt, for example, have a particularly good selection and although alternative and cheaper toy-type versions of several of the items are available elsewhere, we have found that the real thing stands up to wear and tear very well. To start with, the drill bells which consist of two or four bells on a wooden handle are a useful rattle type toy as are the jingle bells which have several small bells on a strip of leather with a wooden handle. The bright red maracas which are made of fairly strong plastic and make a pleasant sort of sifting sound when shaken have been most successful with some children who have shown little interest in other toys at the Toy Library. They are surprisingly light for their size which is also an advantage. Castanets on handles have also been a favourite with some children although the resultant noise has been less popular with adults! The various types of bell, the maracas and the castanets can all be treated in the same way as rattles.

For older babies the tambourine is an interesting toy both visually and auditorily. Make sure you choose one with well fastened bells that are not sharp on the edges. A tambourine can be used for a number of play activities. At first just let the child explore and shake it for himself. If it is too heavy for him you could try suspending it on a piece of string and sitting him directly in front of it. If he shows little interest in handling it, take his hand and show him how to bang on it. This can often develop into a social game where you bang on the tambourine and then wait for the child to have his turn. When he can bang it try scratching on the tambourine and see if he will also imitate this; then shaking the tambourine, and so on.

Skills taught: AUDITORY DISCRIMINATION
                   HAND AND ARM CONTROL
                   IMITATION

Miscellaneous Ideas

All of the following have some value in individual cases: felt and other textured bricks; 'feely' bags made from different types of material and filled with different things such as dried peas, butter beans or lentils; crinkly paper and paper bags; light cardboard boxes and string; lights, for example, shining a torch beam on a dark surface, especially one that you can change the colours of the beam with, or a flashing light on a Pifco Lantern torch, or an oil and water lamp to watch. With stimuli like these that a baby has no control over, use them only when you are there to see what effect they are having and use them in response to the child's reaction. The same is true if you should try tying stirrup bells on a leather strip round your child's wrist. Watch this carefully because although it can sometimes be a useful way to get a very inactive or uninterested child to react, it can upset him if he cannot 'switch it off', that is every time he involuntarily moves his arm the bell rings.

This chapter has covered only a selection of the wide variety of toys now available for babies. You may find many other toys that a baby will be interested in watching but is not yet able to operate on his own — perhaps a music box TV or a bubble blower, for example. Toys of this nature are included in the sections for older children. Many babies, and especially handicapped babies who are slow to start handling toys for themselves, do enjoy and learn from watching older children playing and from adults using household objects. So as soon as a baby is ready, prop him in positions where he can watch things going on.

For some handicapped babies and children who are slow to develop control of their movements or slow to take an interest in play and toys, this can be a difficult time to select suitable playthings. As mentioned before in the section on teaching techniques, you will need to try out a variety of materials to find a few things that will take their interest. In these instances, try and compensate by involving the child in lots of social play.

CHAPTER 4

Toddlers (1-3 Years): Object Related Play

Skills to Develop

(1) Extensive exploratory play – e.g. examining objects, emptying containers, looking into bags.
(2) Constructive play – e.g. stacking beakers, taking bricks in and out of a container, posting shapes.
(3) Manual dexterity – including feeding himself with a spoon.
(4) Crawling and walking.
(5) Understanding of simple instructions.
(6) Imitating adults.
(7) Imaginative play – e.g. pushing car along a surface with appropriate noises, pretending to feed doll.
(8) Talking – single words, then two-word combinations and, finally, short sentences.

This chapter and the next will be relevant to many children who are not yet walking but have acquired most of the skills outlined in the *Babies* section. They will also relate to many children who are older than toddlers in years but still need to learn most or some of the skills listed above.

Playing to Learn

The period 1-3 years in normal play development is characterised at the beginning by extensive exploratory play: literally the 'he's into everything' stage. Things are examined, tried out in various ways, tipped out, opened up, taken apart, shaken, thrown deliberately, pushed, pulled and rolled. Gradually more constructive forms of play also begin to develop. Instead of just scattering a set of nesting beakers around and examining individual ones, the child tries to fit them together or to build them into a tower. His play is beginning to show purpose and an awareness of delayed cause and effect (e.g. 'If I put these pieces on the stick and then press the button they will fly off again'). He starts to use single words meaningfully and by three years can talk in short 3-5 word

44

sentences. He now begins to play pretend-type games where, for example, he runs a car along the pattern in the carpet or feeds a teddy, and later starts to enjoy model play with farms, garages, dolls' houses, etc. and also role play where he pretends to be certain people.

The range of toys and play activities open to him at this stage is obviously enormous so this chapter focuses on certain types or groups of toys which are useful for developing particular skills — although one of the hallmarks of a good toy is that it is flexible and encourages the child to develop skills in several areas. Everyday toys such as teddies, dolls, cars, are not dealt with because they are so familiar and widely available. This is not to say that they should be undervalued as it is important that a child should have toys he simply enjoys without any specifically 'educational' benefit. A child will learn something from any toy he plays with and so any toy could in fact be called an educational toy. On the other hand, if this approach is taken to extremes, a child might learn a lot about nursing dolls or pushing cars but nothing about matching shapes or colours. Fortunately, recent toy design has produced some very interesting yet at the same time educational toys in the traditional sense of the word. There are a wide variety of posting boxes, for instance — some on wheels, some in the shape of houses, one like a cash till with keys to press down, and another in the shape of a teddy bear with a removable hat for a lid. Fisher-Price have brought out an excellent colour matching toy called a cash register which has been a firm favourite in our Toy Library.

Early Fitting Toys

Early fitting toys range from the simple peg and hold type to cars, lorries and trains that can have men or pieces fitted on to them. Straightforward wooden peg and hole type toys can be rather boring but there are some interesting variations with additional activities involved. Two of the best are Tunnel Pegs by ESA (£6) and Pop-up-Toy by Galt (£3.26). The Fisher-Price Clic n'Clatter Car, although not specifically designed as a fitting toy, has a large man with an easily graspable head which fits into a large hole and makes an ideal early fitting toy. Following from this, Escor have a whole range of wooden toys such as boats and cars with wooden men that are also ideal for fitting (see illustration).

Most children can take pieces out of toys long before they start to try and put them back again. This is hardly surprising as it takes a lot more control and careful eye–hand co-ordination to fit a piece back in. Fitting is one area where many handicapped children do need to be helped at first, otherwise they are likely to just give up or throw the pieces. So if you are going to present one of these toys it is a good idea to do it only when you have time to sit down and watch how the child copes with it; if he needs help you can then step in as soon as it becomes apparent.

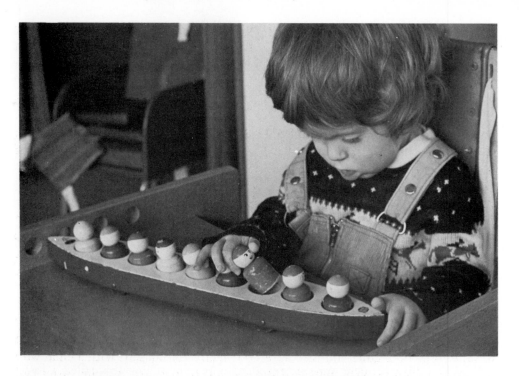

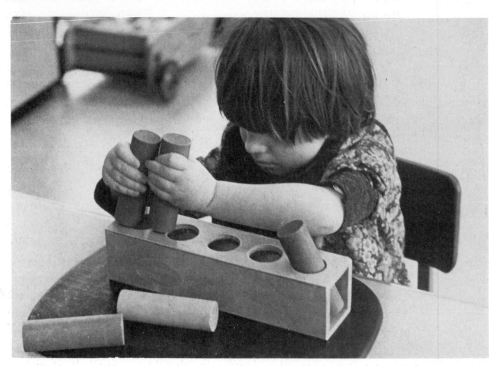

Tunnel Pegs are useful as a first fitting toy although the pegs can be rather large for particularly tiny children. Because the pegs are relatively large and solid this toy is not very suitable for a child who throws frequently unless you intend to supervise his play closely. As well as being fitted into holes the pegs can also be slid through the central 'tunnel' and generally this is the easier thing to start teaching. Wait till the child has had time to examine the toy and roll and bang the pegs, etc. and then demonstrate how the pegs slide through the tunnel. You can make it all the more exciting by having an empty tin or a bowl of water that the pegs land in. If you hold it in front of the child and tilt the tunnel slightly the peg will run through and fall out the other end all in full view of the child. Once you have got his interest and attention you can hand him a peg, point to the opening of the tunnel and see if he will try and 'post' it. Try to hand him the peg in the correct orientation for posting it as an initial problem is often that the child has the peg at the wrong angle to get it in the tunnel. If he makes no attempt to put the peg in the tunnel or is unsuccessful, guide his hand and show him how to do it. If he objects to physical guidance or is reluctant to hold a peg, try holding the peg halfway into the tunnel so all it needs is a push to set it in motion. Once he is able to post the peg when it is handed to him by you, see if he can manage to pick it up off the floor or a table and orientate it correctly for himself. With a child who has poor attention, you may find that he will fit one peg in quite easily and then seem to 'forget' about the rest. Keep it as a game but do encourage him to put them all in so he learns what it is to complete a task and also to pay attention to one activity for longer.

The Pop-up Toy has four wooden pegs with faces painted on one end of each. These pegs bob up and down when tapped because of springs at the bottom of the holes they fit into. (The holes are far too long and narrow for a child to get his finger down and dislodge a spring.)

To start with, as well as encouraging the child to remove the pegs, you can also show him how to bounce the pegs up and down by patting them. If they are patted vigourously enough they will in fact jump out, much to the delight of many children. A more sophisticated way of doing this is to push the peg down with your index finger and suddenly let go so that the peg will bounce out. A surprising number of children learn to do this if you demonstrate it to them a few times. If the child is not well co-ordinated you may need to hold the base still for him or get him to hold it with his other hand as it is fairly easy to knock over.

The four pegs are each painted in a primary colour with a corresponding colour strip running down the side of the toy in front and behind of the hole. Unless the child takes particular notice of the colours it is best to start by treating this primarily as a fitting exercise (although when you demonstrate match the pegs to the correct colour strips) by allowing the child to try and fit any peg into any hole initially. If you need to prompt him to put a peg into a hole guide it to the correct colour if possible. Once he can get the pegs into the holes you can begin teaching colour matching if this has not emerged of its own accord, In fact, although the colour strips run down each side of the toy they do not actually surround the hole at the top. To make things easier for the child we have found it useful to paint the appropriate colour round the hole as many children do not look at the sides. Similarly, to make it easier to colour match you can offer them the pegs face side down so they are simply matching the coloured end of the peg to the coloured hole surround. With most children it will be enough to point at the correct hole and stop them if they start to move towards the wrong hole. You may need to do this many times before the child realises what it is you are requiring him to do, that is before he realises that colour matching is what you are after.

If a child seems unimpressed by fitting toys try the Clic n' Clatter Car. This is an excellent toy in its own right for babies and toddlers, with a ball-shaped wheel at the front which spins round and two large ratcheted red wheels at the back which have indentations for little fingers. All these things make a noise when turned round as does the whole car when run along the floor.

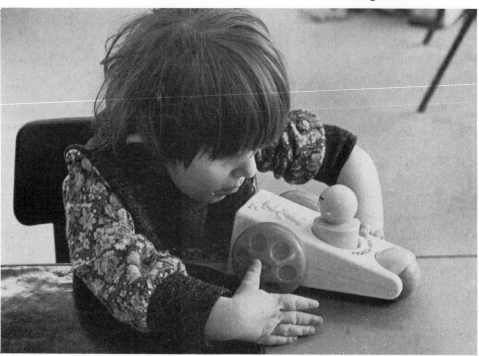

Once a child is used to playing with the Clic n' Clatter Car you can make more of a game of it by jumping the man in and out with a big 'Oo!' and a gasp. If this engages the child's interest take his hand and show him how to jump the man in and out for himself. If this is successful you can progress to the more difficult fitting involved with the Escor toys using similar sorts of games.
Skills taught: EYE–HAND CO-ORDINATION
FINE MOTOR CONTROL

Graded Fitting and Stacking

The next step is where a child not only has to fit something into an appropriate hole or slot but also has to choose the correct size piece for it. This is a much more difficult task and if you watch a young child with a set of nesting beakers you will see that although he is capable of fitting one beaker inside another if given the correct one, he has difficulty in selecting the correct one for himself.

The earliest and most widely available size-grading toys are nesting beakers and variations on them like stacking castles and pile-up pans. Shops like Boots and Mothercare stock versions of these as do many other toy shops. Stacking toys with a central rod that the pieces are fitted on to are also common. Kiddicraft make an attractive one called Rainbow Tree and Fisher-Price have one on a rocking base called Rock-a-stack.

Once a child can put one piece inside another or stack one piece on top of another fairly easily, watch to see if he gets the correct pieces by luck or is beginning to discriminate for himself. If he shows little sign of consistent discrimination start by structuring the material for him. In other words, hand him the pieces in the correct order and encourage him to fit them all together or stack them up. If he has difficulty doing this give as much help as he needs by, for example, taking his hand and showing him how to place one beaker on another. Make this activity into a game where he can knock them all down when they have been built up. King of the Castle, a set of beakers with notched tops like a castle wall and a king who fits on the top is good for these sort of games. It is also very useful for children with poor co-ordination because the notched beakers stack more firmly into each other than ordinary nesting beakers. You may find you need to hold the beaker base still for the child at first (see illustration), but eventually he can be encouraged to hold it with his other hand.

Once he is enjoying playing games when pieces are handed to him in the correct order, you can progress to laying out the pieces for him on the table or floor. Put the first needed piece nearest to him and so on to maximise his chances of getting them in the right order; if he goes to the wrong piece point to the correct one and physically prompt him if necessary. Learning to discriminate one piece from another on the basis of size is much more difficult and you will need to simplify the task by only offering him two very different pieces at first. Present him with the correct piece and another quite different in size and see if he can pick out the right one. Be careful not to place the correct one consistently on the left or the right or he may well pick up the wrong signals and think you are asking him to reach for whatever is on the left (or right). Once he has learnt this first discrimination, gradually introduce pieces that are nearer to the correct one in size and help him at each stage until he is able to discriminate all the pieces correctly. This is a difficult task for some children and they may take a long time to learn these more difficult discriminations. At first use just the biggest, the middle and the smallest nesting beakers.

Skills taught: EYE– HAND CO-ORDINATION
VISUAL SEARCH STRATEGIES
SIZE DISCRIMINATIONS

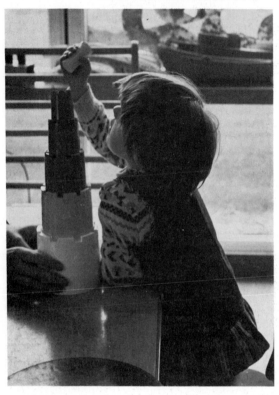

Shape Matching

There is a massive range of shape matching toys on the market from the traditional wooden posting boxes to the till-like Palitoy Shape Register. The advantage of this range is that you can choose a posting box that may suit your child's level of competence and also engage his interest. Some children seem to love playing with the traditional wooden posting boxes whereas others show no interest at all, so it is useful to borrow one to try out first. Their advantage is that they are solidly made and relatively stable for a poorly co-ordinated child to use. They are usually clear and uncluttered in design so that a slow learning child or a child with perceptual or visual problems will find little to confuse him. The shapes also make a satisfying noise as they drop into the box and spares to some makes (ESA, Galt) are available. These boxes are usually strong and have no extra pieces that can be pulled off so they are suitable for children who are destructive with toys and in settings such as nurseries, play schools and special schools where they will get a lot of use. The major drawback is that some handicapped children, in particular, do not find them intrinsically very interesting but this is not necessarily a problem if you plan to use a posting box primarily as a one-to-one teaching toy either at home or at school.

A good example of a simple basic posting box is the Abbat Posting Box by ESA at £2.94. This has a detachable lid and in the Toy Library we have found this sort of design seems to last better than posting boxes with hinged or sliding lids which are more likely to get broken. Unless your child appears to be particularly good at shape matching it is usually better to start with one of these simpler boxes with only three or four basic shapes – circle, triangle, square, narrow oblong – as more shapes will only confuse him and may lead to frustration. Four-to-Eight have produced a set which has both a wooden posting box and a transparent plastic posting box with eight changeable lids with different shapes in them and 39 different posting pieces. It is particularly useful for teaching a child shape discrimination by a number of graded steps and would be of value in a school because it can be used with a range of children. It is well designed as a teaching aid and, at £26.40, falls more into this category than that of 'toy'.

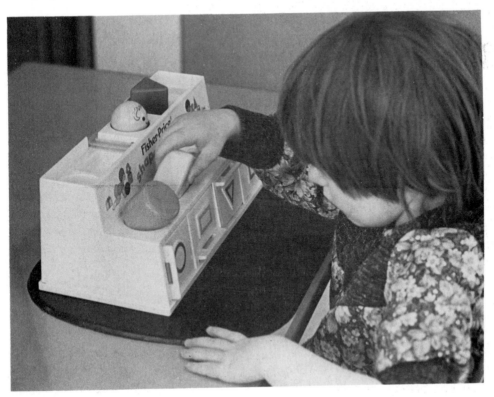

One of the best of the plastic posting boxes for early shape matching is the

Shape Sorter by Fisher-Price. In the accompanying illustration Eileen is playing quite contentedly on her own with a shape sorter. As well as having a tray on top that the four pieces fit into, the sorter has four holes so that each can be posted into its own small compartment with a hinged door for retrieving the piece. Each door is marked with the appropriate shape and opens a different way round to the other doors. There is also a little round head on the top which squeaks when pressed. This toy is high in intrinsic interest for most children and ideal for a child like Eileen who enjoys active exploratory play and is just starting to play constructively. Another advantage is that like many of the wooden posting boxes this has a broad base which helps to make it more stable. Notice that Eileen's teacher has put a non-slip mat underneath so it will not slide around the table, and has cleared the table of any other distractions.

A useful and relatively inexpensive plastic posting box in the shape of a real post box is the one made by Kiddicraft. Many versions of this exist and Orchard toys have recently brought out a posting bucket along similar lines. These are popular with children for carrying around and filling and emptying with a whole variety of objects. Some of them are not as stable as the previously mentioned posting boxes and are therefore less suitable for poorly co-ordinated children.

There are some interesting variations on these basic posting boxes. Susan Wynter Toys, for example, have produced a wooden posting house. This has a vary wide base and a sloping top so it is easy to use in bed or on a table. It is designed so the pieces automatically return and the holes are an integral part of the picture of a house. Playskool have recently brought out a very attractive posting teddy bear in bright clear plastic (see photographs on p. 17). The pieces are posted into the body of the bear and retrieved by taking his hat-cum-lid off. There is a squeaker on top of his hat and the hat is attached to his body by a length of plastic. The bear has to be rotated to find the correct hole and there are six pieces so this is probably best used with children after they have had some experience with a more basic posting box.

Another posting toy that has to be rotated to find the correct slot is the Tupperware posting ball. This also involves a lot more shapes which are retrieved by holding a handle on either side of the ball and pulling it apart so all the shapes drop out. Posting boxes on wheels are popular and tend to take a child's interest more readily than a static posting box, the only problem being that they may play with it in other ways but never post any shapes unless encouraged to do so. One well liked in the Toy Library is the Royal Mail Post Van by Galt which can also be used as a pull-along. It has a sliding door at the back so that pieces can be taken in and out and is made of wood. Mothercare have a similar toy in bright plastic called a play fit Pull-a-Long Truck with pieces that can be posted in and a driver who bobs up and down when it is pulled along. When choosing a posting toy you have to weigh the value of having novel attention-getting extras against the additional confusion and distraction they might cause for a slow learning child. Probably the best guideline is to go for interest if you want a toy that will amuse a child and that he can play with in some way on his own, and go for a more distraction free toy if you want to use it specifically to teach him shape matching. The ideal toy will vary from child to child but toys like the Tupperware ball and Fisher-Price Shape Sorter probably come closest to this.

Another more complicated shape matching toy that centres interest extremely well is the Palitoy Shape Register. This has eight shapes that are fitted into slots on top of the register. The key with the corresponding shape picture on it has to be depressed in order for the shape to fall into the till. By turning the handle at the side of the till the drawer can be sprung open and the shapes retrieved. This toy is not suitable for very rough or destructive treatment as the shapes can be rammed through the slots without pressing the keys with the result that it gets jammed up and the mechanisms inside are broken. If it is given to a child who is taught to use it properly, or is unlikely to use force, it is a very good toy with a great deal of intrinsic interest and a lot of teaching value both with an adult and for a child playing on his own. It is important to remember that many shape matching toys, like fitting toys, are spectacularly unsuccessful if just dumped on a young handicapped child without any help or guidance. They can easily lead to frustration and rejection or to total lack of interest very quickly, which means only introducing them when you have time to sit down and show the child what to do.

Many children enjoy taking the lid off posting toys and putting various objects including the shapes into the box and emptying them out but do not show any signs of spontaneously trying to post the pieces through their appropriate holes. It may be useful to let a child have one or two other toys with lids like plastic saucepans or beakers that he can fill and empty and keep the posting box initially for teaching shape matching.

Shape matching really involves two basic sets of skills:

being able to fit the shapes into the slots;
knowing which shape goes into which slot.

Nearly all children can discriminate and fit the round shape before any of the others, especially if the round one is a ball rather than a round peg (as in the Galt posting box). In fact if a child is having difficulties posting pieces to start with it is worth substituting a wooden ball for a wooden peg if you can find one of the right size. The advantage of the ball is that it will fit in any way round and does not have to be correctly orientated. Once the child can cope with a ball he can progress to using a rounded peg, handed to him in the correct orientation. If it seems a difficult skill for the child to learn it is often better to simplify the task and teach the fitting and the discrimination as two separate steps. You can start by handing a child a shape and pointing or, if necessary, guiding his hand to the right hole. Once he can post the four basic shapes when they are handed to him, you can put them on the table or floor to see if he can orientate them correctly for himself. Some children enjoy posting, others obviously find it of little interest. If the child you are dealing with falls into the second category try to turn it into an interesting game for him. For example, you could circle your hand round slowly and then suddenly pop a shape in; you can reward him with lots of praise or a sip of drink or whatever he enjoys when he has successfully dropped in the shape, even if you have helped him. Posting toys that have the built-in reward of the child wanting to do whatever comes next are useful from this point of view, like putting pieces in the Fisher-Price shape sorter so he can have the reward of opening the doors and taking them out.

You may find that he has learnt to pick the correct hole for each shape in the process of being taught to post them; if not, guide his hand to the correct hole, starting with the circle as this is the easiest. Do not forget to turn the box round between goes or he might simply learn always to go for the bottom right hand corner! Sometimes tapping by the hole you want him to post into is useful with a child who is not really attending. Next carry out the same process with the square. Then give him the square and the circle alternately to see if he can switch between searching for one then the other. Give a prompting point or physical guidance if he starts to go wrong but do not let him become entirely dependent on you helping him. Carry on with this process until he is able to post all four shapes successfully, before introducing more complex posting with more shapes and factors like having to turn the box to find the correct shape. As before teach this step by step and try not to let him flounder. Eileen, for example, although able to cope with the shape sorter on her own, needed a lot of guidance from her teacher on turning the posting bear to find the correct hole for each shape. As with the early fitting toys, if the child shows great reluctance to hold the pieces even, start by holding them over the correct slot yourself and encourage him to give them a push so they drop into the box.

With the Palitoy shape register you will have to teach the child not only to match the shapes to their slots but also to the pictures on the keys. Some mothers have found it useful actually to take the shape the child has put in a slot and hold it by each of the keys until he spots the correct picture, and then put it back in the slot ready for him to press the correct key. If the child is not ready to do this and shows no sign of recognising the correct picture, despite help, let him put all the shapes in and then by pressing all the keys he will get all the shapes into the drawer. This is a useful toy for helping a child to learn a sequence of events that must be performed in a particular order. It does not really matter where he starts in the sequence: the important thing is to teach him all the stages and take him through it several times gradually withdrawing help as he learns to do more of it himself. You might have the following sequence, for example, which starts with shapes in the till and the drawer closed.

(1) Pull handle to open drawer.

(2) Take shapes out and put on floor.
(3) Close drawer.
(4) Put shapes into slots.
(5) Press keys.

Most of the steps cannot be performed until the step before is performed so it helps impose an ordered sequence on the child. Some children left to their own devices tend to play with the toy in a random trial-and-error fashion, and although they spend a lot of time looking very busy, if you watch closely they are often being very repetitive and may spend 15 minutes or so just opening and closing the drawer, for instance. In this case try and encourage them to go through the whole sequence so they are learning to structure their play and use a number of skills.

One final tip: some posting boxes have at least one set of spare shapes. It is a good idea to remove these as (a) they can cause confusion, and (b) you can replace any of the first set should they get lost.

Skills taught: EYE–HAND CO-ORDINATION
DISCRIMINATION OF SIZE
SEARCH STRATEGIES AND SEQUENCING

Table 4.1: Popular Posting Boxes

Toy	Supplier or Manufacturer	Obtainable & Price
Cube Posting Box (3 sets of shapes with hinged lid)	Galt	Galt catalogue and shops. Better toy shops. (£4.30)
Abbatt Posting Box (fitted lid, 2 sets of shapes, wooden)	ESA	ESA catalogue. Better toy shops. (£2.94)
Shape Sorter	Fisher-Price	Generally available.
Posting box (plastic)	Kiddicraft and others	Generally available.
Posting Bear	Playskool	Some shops.
Posting Bucket	Orchard Toys	Some shops.
Tupperware Ball	Tupperware	Tupperware agents.
Royal Mail Post Van (pull-along)	Galt	Galt catalogue and shops. (£8.75)
Posting House (wooden)	Susan Wynter	Susan Wynter catalogue. (£5)
Play Fit pull-along Truck	Mothercare	Mothercare shops or catalogue. (£5.65)

Colour Matching

The average child can match two or three primary colours by the time he is three years old. There is a lot of variation in the development of a skill like this but many toys that are useful for colour matching can be used in other ways first so that often a child starts to colour match spontaneously without ever being shown. One thing that has to be realised is that the child has to 'know' that the purpose of the toy is to colour match. He may be able to sort yellow and red bricks out into two separate piles of his own accord but not match the Galt pop-up-men to the correct slots because he either does not know or does not choose to colour match. Children who are generally slow in learning are less likely to start colour matching spontaneously so toys and games can be used to encourage it. There are quite a few toys produced specifically for this purpose and others where colour matching is not the only or the primary skill that the toy is designed to teach. The 'climbing clowns', for example, although not produced as a colour matching toy, do in fact fulfil this role very well. The Galt pop-up-men already mentioned under 'fitting' toys are another useful early colour matching toy. Colour matching is, of course, different from colour labelling, where the child can name colours correctly, and matching usually occurs before labelling. Escor produce various abacuses which consist of four or five sticks on a base with wooden balls of different colours that can be threaded on to them to match the colour painted on the top of each stick. This is a versatile toy that can be used by younger children merely for taking the balls off; at a later stage they can learn to thread the balls back on and then it can be used for colour matching and eventually counting.

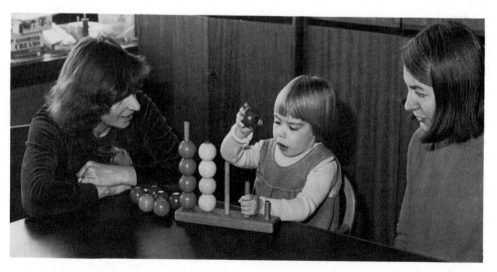

One advantage of the Escor colour matching abacus is that you can just use two colours to start with if necessary. Remove the other colour balls and simply cover the spare rods with your hand. Put one ball on to each of the remaining rods and then point or guide the child with the rest of the balls to the correct rod. Make sure he is seated so that he can comfortably reach the top of the rods otherwise you may need to tilt them towards him. If he has difficulty fitting them on it may be because he tries to put the ball on without realising he has to line up the hole in the ball with the rod. Point to the hole and when you guide his hand make sure he is looking as you line up the hole and peg. This is quite a difficult perceptual task but some children have found a neat solution to it. They put their index finger right through the hole in the ball and then the tip of their finger on top of the rod. By straightening up their finger which is like an extension of the rod they can get the ball to slide off and down the rod. Although you cannot demonstrate this (an adult's finger is too large) I have sometimes put a ball on a child's finger and then placed their finger on top of a rod.

Early colour matching toys should involve no more than three or four primary colours and any items that come in sets of a few clear colours can be used. To start off with you could lay out a large red and a large yellow nesting beaker then give the child a small red beaker and see if he can put it in or on the right one. Similarly, with the climbing clowns, you could put one yellow and one red clown on the base, hand him a red or yellow clown, and see if he can put it on the same colour clown. You may have to demonstrate this several times and point or physically guide the child to the correct one until he realises you want him to colour match. It is no good just *saying* 'Put it on the red one' as the labelling may have very little meaning for him at this stage. Using bits and pieces of toys like this rather than a specific colour matching toy is useful at first because it is easier to begin with just two colours. Many children learn to match red and yellow most easily of the primary colours but have more difficulty discriminating between and correctly matching blue, red and green. For this reason and to cut down on confusion, start with two colours (preferably red and yellow) and only introduce a third when the child can reliably match the first two. Prompt him as soon as he *starts* to go wrong if you suspect he has little idea about what is required or you may just confuse and frustrate him if, for example, you make him move his clown from the top of one clown to another. Although the relevant cue to attend to may be obvious to you it may not be at all obvious to a toddler. Going off cue is a constant problem with children until their understanding of language is good enough to follow quite complicated verbal instructions. Toys like the climbing clowns which are the same shape and size, help to focus the child on the *colour* cue: the child is not tempted to match them by shape and size. Make sure also that the child is really attending to the task. I remember one occasion working on shape matching with a little Down's syndrome girl. I was feeling rather pleased with myself as she was matching the square to the correct slot every time. But then I realised she was watching my face carefully each time she picked the square up and started to move it towards one end of the board; if she saw me smile she knew she was going towards the correct slot and carried on, whereas if I gave no response she realised she was wrong and changed direction — intelligent behaviour on her part but she was not attending to the task and certainly was not learning much about shape matching!

As with shape matching, colour matching toys that have a lot of intrinsic interest are especially useful. One of the 'top ten' in the Toy Library this year has definitely been the Fisher-Price Cash Register. This has three different colour discs that have to be put in the slots with the matching key colours to the discs. The discs are slightly different sizes so they will only disappear when the key is pressed if they have been matched to the correct slot. If the green button at the side is pressed the discs disappear into the drawer, and if the orange button is pressed they run back down the change shute. Like the Shapes Register this is good for teaching a child a sequence of activities and can, of course, be used for imaginative play. It also has the advantage of only introducing three primary colours. The one drawback with slow learning children is that colour matching the key and the slot is not obvious because of the gap between them. In fact it is worth sticking matching bright coloured tape from the top of the key to the slot to make the colour matching more clear cut and obvious. Despite this it is an excellent toy because of the amount of enjoyment many children get out of it and the variety of activities involved.

It is often a good idea to start by putting the discs into the correct slots yourself and getting the child to press the keys to make the discs disappear. If you put in just one disc at a time you can observe whether your child realises he needs to press the key directly below the slot to get the disc to drop in or if he just presses the keys in random order. If the latter is true, prompt by pointing or physically guiding his hand to the correct key. As with most toys it is probably best to demonstrate all of the activities on it and then give him a chance to show which he can do on his own. You will then be in a position to know what he needs help with (such as opening the drawer or pressing the side keys to make the discs drop). If he can manage most of the activities but is haphazard in his approach and rarely goes through the whole sequence try to prompt him to do so by pointing or drawing his attention to the next thing he needs to do. Two sets of discs are supplied and as with some of the posting boxes it saves confusion and provides spares if you keep one set in reserve.

Skills taught: COLOUR MATCHING AND DISCRIMINATION
                  SEARCH STRATEGIES AND SEQUENCING

Constructional and Building Toys

Constructional toys is a fairly loose term to cover a variety of toys where anything from several pieces up to a few hundred are put together to make a

structure of some sort. At this early stage only simpler building and constructional toys will be dealt with. The earliest of these are things like bricks or
nesting beakers that can be piled on top of one another to build a tower (see
p. 50). A set of small (1-2 inch) bricks in a trolley for taking in and out and
later stacking up (wooden are generally better than plastic for this) are a
traditional toy and widely available. On the whole they are not particularly
useful for younger handicapped children probably because they lack intrinsic
interest and need the child to bring imagination and interest to them. On the
other hand very large house-brick-size plastic bricks that lock easily together
are popular. They are called Lincabricks and are available from Galt in sets
of 24 at £13 per set.

Early constructional toys need to be easy to fit together and to have pieces
that can be fitted in any order so that success is virtually guaranteed. A toy
that we have found very successful and that has these requirements is 'climbing
clowns', mentioned in the previous section. These are fairly widely available
and are best if you can get them with a base in the form of a plastic pull-along
truck. They consist of a number of square-shaped hollow plastic men nearly
three inches high that fit on top of each other. They can also be fitted by
rounded arms to semicircles at the bottom of their bodies but this requires
more skill and is not usually introduced till some time after the child can
stack them. The clowns are ideal for inventing a lot of fun games so they are
not simply seen as a stacking task for the child. You can run them up to the
truck and then jump one on to the base of the truck and then the next one on
to the head of the first one and so on. Many children are delighted with this
and are keen to imitate for themselves.

Kiddicraft make a toy called a Floot-a-toota which consists of about twelve
pieces that fit together to make a long plastic trumpet. This can be blown to
produce various sounds. If you start the trumpet off for the child, then hand
him the next piece and point or help him fit it, and carry on until the whole
trumpet is made, this is often quite successful. If he enjoys blowing down the
trumpet it means the reward is built in for him. If he is poor at fitting the
pieces on or gets impatient easily, start by getting him to fit only one piece
on and then let him have a blow and gradually increase the number of pieces
he has to fit on.

Another simple constructional toy by Kiddicraft is called Curly Coiler. This
is a snake which is made by snapping together a head, a tail and nine body
sections. Use the same sort of teaching technique as for the Floot-a-toota.

Skills taught: EYE–HAND CO-ORDINATION
                   CONSTRUCTIVE PLAY

Early Screwing, Threading and Joining Toys

These sort of toys are often mentioned in conjunction with encouraging fine motor co-ordination. While it is true that handling many toys requires the precise and skilful use of the hand and fingers, the sort of toys described below place particularly high demands on the child's ability to make fine motor adjustments and also require him to use both hands in a co-ordinated manner. Many toys of this type exist but are often rather dull and some are better viewed as educational teaching aids. A few of the more interesting ones have been picked out for discussion here.

Threading Probably the best set of early threading beads that can be found at present are the big translucent solid plastic ones by ESA. These are very eye catching and attractive when the light shines through them and do make a good toy for stringing across a baby's cot or for encouraging visual tracking (see illustration). The beads are just over an inch long and an inch wide — an ideal size for small hands and the stiff plastic thread is also easy to handle. The average child would probably start threading between two and three years of age.

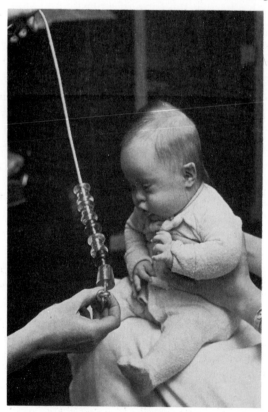

Let the child play with the beads and the thread for a while and then demonstrate how to thread the beads on. If you need to get his attention thread the bead on with the thread held high up so that the bead holds his attention as it rushes down. Once he is interested, give him the thread with about an inch poking out of his hand and put the bead with one of the holes facing towards the thread in his other hand and see if he can thread it for himself. If not, guide just one hand if possible, or both if necessary. The difficult bit is often teaching children that once they have threaded the bead they must then use that hand to take hold of the thread now poking out of the bead, and then let go with the other hand so the bead can slide down the thread. Quite often they fail to grab hold of the thread and the beads drop off again. This is quite a complicated sequence for a child to learn so guide him in easy stages: you may find you need to hold the thread for him to start with while he threads the bead on; alternatively, you must be ready to grab hold of the thread when he manages to get it through the bead. Once he can thread the beads you can play simple colour matching games where you encourage him to choose all the blue beads to thread on, or all the red beads, and so on.

Screwing This is a difficult skill for some children to learn and whereas the average child seems to pick it up from being shown how to unscrew the odd top off a jar or piece off a toy, some children seem to need more practice at it and in these cases toys designed specifically to do this can be helpful.

An old favourite is 'Billie and his Barrels' by Kiddicraft; it is also produced under other names. There are six barrels, each in two halves that screw together, and graded in size so they fit inside each other, and fixed inside the smallest barrel is a little plastic man. Unscrewing the barrels is easier than screwing them up again which involves aligning the two halves precisely. Some children with very tiny hands may not be able to manage the larger barrels even to undo. Start with the barrels very loosely screwed together so that the slightest turn will unscew them. If your child has developed right or left handedness, take his non-preferred hand (i.e. the hand he uses less often) and place one half of the barrel in it. Take his other hand and place it over the other half of the barrel and prompt him to twist his hand until the barrel is unscrewed. The barrels inside at this stage usually fall on the floor so you will have to remind him to put down the two halves he is holding and pick up the rest. Repeat the process until you get to 'Billie'. If you have the barrels a little more firmly screwed together you will have to show him that after each twist he needs to replace his hands and twist again from the centre until the barrel is unscrewed. If your child is not very impressed with finding Billie in the middle of the barrel try a small sweet like a smartie. Again if his patience and attention span are poor, cut down the number of barrels to begin with although, surprisingly perhaps, many children do enjoy the anticipation and excitement of going through all the barrels.

Screwing the barrels back together also involves the task of selecting two halves of the same size. Make things easier at first by handing him the correct halves or having them placed in pairs ready for him. If he can colour match he can pick out the correct half either by size or colour, colour probably being easier overall. If you want him to select the correct half by *size*, present him with one of the largest and one of the smallest barrels to make it easier for him.

Various screwing rods are also available. Galt have a straightforward one with a central plastic rod and lots of plastic nuts that can be screwed on and off it. Kiddicraft have produced a useful one called 'Twist n' Turn' which has three very large different shaped pieces that can be screwed on and off. You can either get the child to unscrew the nuts using a similar technique to that used with the barrels or, if he is poorly co-ordinated, you can begin by just spinning the pieces off. With rods like the Galt rod which are fairly long, make sure he holds it in the middle or nearer to the end he is using otherwise he will not have enough control over it. For spinning the pieces off, instead of having to prompt him to hold the nut with his individual fingers, you can show him how to use his fingers as a body to stroke downwards or upwards on the nut and spin it off this way. As with the barrels, start with the nut right at the end of the rod so the slightest spin will get it off. Some children learn to use just their index finger to do this. You should try and make whatever you demonstrate as interesting as possible so he will want to copy. Spin the nuts off the rod suddenly, for example, or exclaim with surprise when you find Billy in the middle of the barrels.

For finer finger control, the Escor constructional toys, like the two horse roundabout, are ideal because they all have four-pronged plastic wing nuts holding the various pieces together (spare nuts are available). Small plastic jars with plastic lids with things hidden inside can also make interesting toys, and once he can screw and unscrew you can make it an integral part of his play and everyday activities, such as letting him unscrew the lid on the plastic storage jar where the biscuits are kept.

Joining Fisher-Price have produced some large plastic popper beads that fit together. These are particularly good for encouraging eye–hand co-ordination as the popper part of the bead has to be carefully aligned with the hole on the next bead so thay can be snapped together. The child also has to realise that he needs to have the end of the bead with the hole ready to fit the popper into.

Start by showing the child how to pull the beads apart. If he is not able to do this for himself, place a hand on each of two adjacent beads and prompt him to pull them. When he can do this demonstrate how to pop two beads together. Hand him the two beads in the correct orientation and see if he can do it for himself. Some children find it easier to start with the beads on a table so that they are supported in sliding them together — this requires less motor control than holding them in mid-air. Some children retain their hold on the first bead and do not realise that they need to hold the second one instead when they are preparing to join a third bead on. This is quite a common mistake and you may need to prompt the child to move his hand several times before he catches on. Once he is popping the beads together start leaving the rest on the table so he has to pick them up, look for the hole and turn the bead round himself. Be ready to offer help if he needs it. It is a difficult task requiring a level of concentration, and may take several sessions to learn, so give plenty of praise and encouragement, with clapping, etc. and, if necessary, other rewards such as a drink or a sweet. Do not forget to give these immediately and every time he does something appropriate, even if you are guiding his hands.

Skills taught: EYE–HAND CO-ORDINATION
FINE MOTOR CONTROL
PLANNING AND SEQUENCING ACTIVITY

Surprise Toys

Many of these toys could also be called cause-and-effect toys because the child learns that if he does something like pressing a button something else will happen as a result. Often it is something sudden and exciting hence the 'surprise' element. Most of these toys could be put in some other category as well, such as stacking toys or fitting toys, but their distinguishing feature is that something else happens as a result of what the child does. They are particularly attractive and exciting to most children as quite often the child gets a big response or reward from the toy for relatively little input. This makes them ideal toys for children who are unskilful or uninterested in play and have little imagination and persistence to bring to the play situation.

Pop-up Toys

The pop-up cone or 'Trigger Jigger' is one of the most widely available and popular of these toys. It can be bought in Mothercare, Boots and most toy shops and at around £2.30 is considerably cheaper than many other surprise toys. The spring inside does tend to break if it is subjected to particularly rough and inappropriate play; this is a problem with most surprise toys as there is invariably some mechanism involved making the toy more vulnerable to breakage if treated roughly or destructively. The pop-up cone illustrates one of the advantages of the surprise toy in that a task like threading the cones on, which on a static toy may be of little interest to a child is made worthwhile by the event that follows. This element of having a built-in reward is one of the great assets of using these toys with handicapped children. Another advantage is that once the child has learned what to do he will be able to play with it on its own and not only when he is given adult praise and encouragement.

Other toys based on the same principle as the pop-up cone are also available. Pedigree have produced an attractive Pop-up Humpty Dumpty consisting of six pieces that fly off when the trigger is pressed. This toy is particularly good for children who can recognise Humpty Dumpty and get excitement out of his demise, but on the other hand it is harder to assemble than the pop-up cone as the pieces need to be put on in the correct order and it is more of a nuisance if one of the pieces gets lost. Another toy of this type is the Pop-up Rocket by Kiddicraft. This is well designed in principle but those we have had in the Toy Library so far have had rather badly fitting pieces which have made them frustrating and difficult to stack. We may have had a bad batch but if you can try out the fit of the piece before buying one, do so.

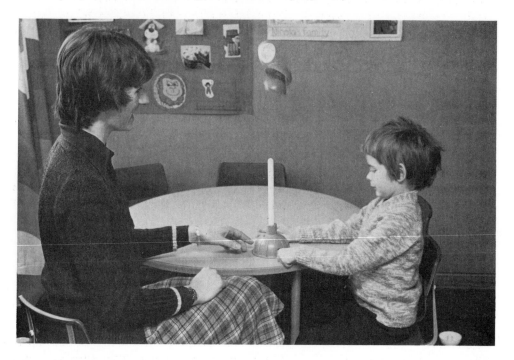

With all these toys demonstrate them to the child a few times and let him examine the toy and the pieces. You can build in extra excitement by things like jumping the spaceman along the ground and up into the nose cone of the rocket and then counting one, two, three before firing it, or with the pop-up cone catching the pieces after they are fired. It does not matter much where-abouts in the sequence you start getting the child to join in if he has not done so spontaneously. Usually pressing the lever or button to fire the toy is the easiest part to teach and has the added advantage of immediate reward. If necessary, take his hand and physically guide him to do this until he can do it on his own. Some children, although excited, are rather apprehensive of firing the toy, especially the pop-up rocket that makes a rather alarming thwack. If this is the case it may be better to start somewhere else in the sequence. With children who tend to be jumpy and nervous of new things you can present these surprise toys at some distance at first and gradually bring them closer as the child gets used to them.

If you think your child is capable of learning the whole sequence fairly quickly it is a good idea to teach him to do all the stages on each go, taking his hand and guiding him or pointing to things for him until he can manage without any help. For example, with the pop-up cone hand him one of the cones and help him thread it on. It is often the case that a child will start to pick the cones up quite willingly but then have difficulty in actually getting them to fit on to the rod, and so become discouraged. Sometimes leaning the rod towards the child helps, especially if he is seated at a table and cannot really see the top of it properly. When he has fired all the pieces off encourage him to pick them all up as children often seem to pick up one or two pieces and 'forget' the rest, even when they are visible.

The pop-up rocket is an ideal toy for breaking the teaching down into stages if necessary. Once a child can fire the rocket you can build the whole rocket up, put the spaceman in and just help him put the nose-cone on. When he can do this you can help him to fit the spaceman in and the nose-cone on, and so on, until he can build up the whole rocket for himself starting from the base. Then you can teach him to press the white firing rod down before building up the rocket at which stage he is able to operate the whole toy for himself. This is called *chaining* and is a useful technique to use whenever you have to teach a child something that can be broken down into a number of distinct stages.

Jack-in-the-boxes

Another extremely successful surprise toy is the Jack-in-the-box. Probably the most robust and easiest to use is the one by Fisher-Price (see illustration). One or two children have been known to break the lid off its hinges but on the whole it stands up very well to quite rough treatment. The warning about introducing surprise toys gradually to some children is very relevant here as the Jack-in-the-box emerges with a hideous squeak which 'frightens the life' out of some children unless they are given time to get used to it. The Jack-in-the-box is released by pushing a button, and a lever at the front can be pressed up and down to make his mouth open and close and eyes rotate. He has to be pushed back in by hand and the lid pressed down ready to start again.

Other Jack-in-the-boxes that play a tune when the handle is turned, terminating in it jumping out, are discussed under musical toys.

As with the pop-up toys the easiest part to teach the child to do is to press the button. If his co-ordination is very poor you can get him to do this with a fisted hand but with physical guidance it is often possible to get a child to press it with his index finger. This is useful as it is not possible to operate the inset lever that makes the mouth move with a fisted hand so he needs to know how to use one or two fingers to press it. Teaching a child to get the Jack-in-the-box back and the lid shut is rather more difficult as it requires good co-ordination

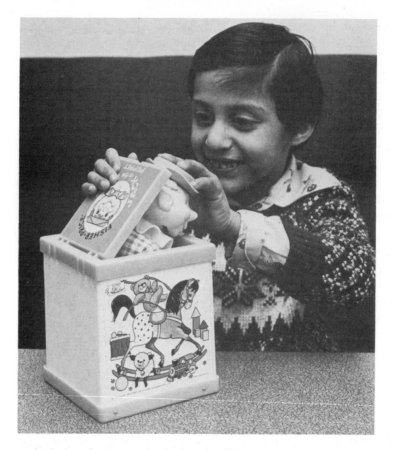

and timing between both hands. First you can get him used to pressing the Jack-in-the-box up and down which many children enjoy as it produces a lot of squeaking. Then prompt him to bring the lid over with his other hand while the first hand is holding the Jack-in-the-box down. The difficult bit is that you have to carry on pressing the lid down with one hand while you time withdrawal of the other hand so that Jack-in-the-box will not pop out again — quite a sophisticated manoeuvre which implies a good understanding of the relationship between the movements of the two parts. It is surprising how many children with a mixture of persistence and force manage to get it back in the box, which is probably some indication of the interest and motivation that a really exciting toy can engender. One note of caution: two or more children often want to play with this toy at the same time, and we have had one or two instances of trapped fingers where one child has pushed the lid down while the other was trying to hold the Jack-in-the-box in. So if your handicapped child is either overwhelmed by brothers and sisters at home or playmates at school, try and find a time or a place where he can have this toy to himself to start with. Surprise toys, in particular, because of their popularity tend to be eagerly fought over, and the handicapped child may not get a look in or may find his play severely disrupted. There is also the additional problem that it is often during these tussles that the toy gets broken.

Frisky Frog and other Squeeze-bulb Toys

There are several toys available that work on the principle of a bulb being squeezed to activate the toy. They all tend to suffer from the problem that the plastic tube joining the bulb to the toy is vulnerable to breakage or detachment from the body of the toy, but if used appropriately this should not happen. The bulbs on some toys tend to be rather stiff so if you know your child has a weak grip try to choose one with a reasonably soft bulb. As well as being good for encouraging finger and hand movement these toys are also good for language and social play. In fact I have sometimes used one of these toys with children who cannot operate them as part of language games planned to encourage either understanding or usage of words like 'stop', 'go', 'jump', 'fall', etc.

Demonstrate the toy and get your child's attention. Quite often children will watch the toy with fascination but not notice or connect the squeezing of the bulb with it. Hold the bulb out in front of them and exaggerate your squeezing to draw their attention to it. After a few goes hand him the bulb and if he does not spontaneously squeeze it, cover his hand with your own and show him how to squeeze. Some children do not seem to have the strength to do this and develop interesting but effective alternatives of their own. Quite a few hit it with a clenched fist; one child I know used to squeeze it with the heel of his foot and another used to put it behind her knee and bend her knee to squeeze it! So if hand squeezing is not successful see if some alternative method will work.

Some children succeed in squeezing the bulb but do not look to see or notice that it is operating the toy. Try and place the toy in their line of vision and direct their attention to it when it moves. Rapid alternating of attention from one object or person to another object or person is something that slow learning children often find difficult to do so this will provide good practice.

Press Button Toys

These toys have several buttons that each operate a different activity. On one called 'Farmer Giles', for example, when the various keys are pressed a duck comes out of a barn, a squawking rooster emerges, a pig comes out of his sty, a cow from a trough and a tractor rolls down a ramp. The large square keys each have a picture of the thing they set in motion, so the child can learn to select a particular one either by picture or spatial position of the button. Another press button toy is in the shape of a tree with a squeaking owl and a tiger that emerges from the top, a squirrel and a pig that emerge from doors and a bear that beats a drum.

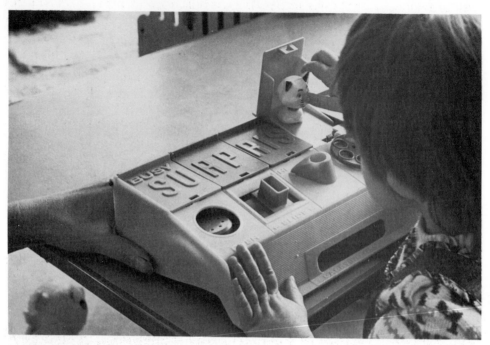

The Surprise Box, or 'Walt Disney Popping Pals' as it is now known, is an excellent although not very robust toy. Each knob is operated in a different manner by pushing, sliding, turning, etc. to release a lid with its attached character (see illustration). If the child is poorly co-ordinated you may need to hold the toy for him if it is likely to topple over or shift around the table, but let him press the keys. Comment and exclaim as the various animals and objects come out as these toys are useful for early language stimulation. This is particularly important with children who play with the toy in a repetitive and stereotyped manner — hitting one key over and over again, for example. Some children can be left to get on with it themselves once they have learned how to press the keys, but with a child who tends to get bored easily and is destructive in consequence, it is best not to leave him too long on his own. Having said this they are fascinating toys for many children and are played with quite happily for hours.

Skills taught: HAND AND FINGER CONTROL
SWITCHING ATTENTION
CAUSE AND EFFECT

Musical Toys

There is a wide range of musical toys available from simple music boxes to quite elaborate musical slides and record players. Many of these toys could also come under other categories such as surprise toys or fitting toys and this is one of the assets of a good musical toy that it does involve the child in several activities. Musical toys have the same sort of advantages and disadvantages as surprise toys in that they are often very attractive to the child who will work hard to operate the toy for the resultant music; but again, like surprise toys, they suffer from the drawback that as a mechanism is usually involved they are also more likely to get broken.

Some of the simplest and most robust of the music box type are the musical radios by Fisher-Price. They play a complete tune like 'Pop goes the Weasel' when fully wound. One problem with all the Fisher-Price musical toys is that the knobs are rather stiff for some children to turn, but high interest and motivation often seems to overcome this. The radio is a fairly limited toy in that it only involves the one activity of winding it up but it is a useful toy to try with children who are difficult to motivate and one that many children get a lot of enjoyment from. Because it is so strong and straightforward to use it is a good toy to give a child to play with on his own once he can wind it for himself. The plastic handle means that it can also be tied to something to prevent its being thrown if this seems advisable.

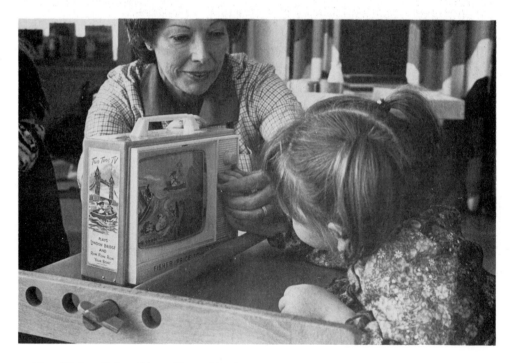

The Fisher-Price 'Two Tune Music Box TV', like the radio, is fairly limited in activity but high in interest and enjoyment. It is a firm favourite with some handicapped children and useful in that they can be left to play with it on their own. In the illustration Karen is being shown how to turn the knob. The

TV is rather more expensive than the radio but of course there is the added fascination of watching the large picture move across the screen.

Various battery operated toy organs are available. One of the most fascinating of these is the 'Big Mouth Singers' by Palitoy. (They also used to produce a similar 'Wombles Piano' that is still sometimes available in shops.) The singers are an excellent toy for a child with limited skills and imagination because for a small amount of effort he can make a lot happen and get a lot of fun. There are eight singers' heads in different colours on top of the organ. Each time a key is pressed a note is played and one of the singers opens his mouth. We have found this toy popular with many children but of particular value with those who have shown little overall interest in toys in general and slow progress in using them. The keys are large and easy to hit even by a child with poor co-ordination; it also involves the child in more activity as he has to hit a key each time he wants to produce a noise and see a singer open his mouth. A colour is blocked in above each key corresponding to one of the singers in colour so that the toy can be used for colour matching as well. The singers are rather vulnerable to attack by smash-and-grab type children so if you think this is likely to be a serious problem it may be better to get a plain plastic organ without any embellishments.

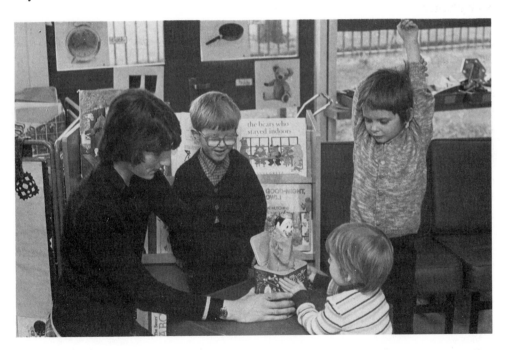

Simple music boxes with handles to wind them up are sometimes fragile and do not stand up to rough treatment too well. They can also be rather frustrating for children who are not able to turn the handle fairly rapidly and continuously, which is necessary in order to obtain a recognisable tune. More successful are the musical Jack-in-the-boxes which play a tune when a handle is turned. Two of the nicest of these are the Burbank Jack-in-the-box and the Kermit Jack-in-the-box. The Burbank one in metal is like a traditional music box in that you turn a handle with a wooden knob to play a tune. At the end the Jack flies out and like the Fisher-Price one then has to be pushed back in and the lid closed. The plastic Kermit one also plays a tune when the handle is turned but at the end with a mighty springing noise two tiers of boxes with a Kermit at the top fly out. The illustration shows the children taking turns to operate the Burbank Jack-in-the-box.

As with some of the surprise toys you should introduce the Jack-in-the-boxes gently (especially the Kermit one). With the music boxes that play a tune as the handle is turned you may need to prompt the child to keep going if he needs to turn it several times before the Jack-in-the-box comes out. With children who tend to give up easily, you may need to play through most of the tune yourself so they just have to do the last little bit. You can then gradually increase the amount of handle turning they do on subsequent occasions.

Xylophones

It is worth getting a reasonably well designed xylophone as the cheaper ones tend to fall apart and the keys are not very securely attached. For children who have reached the banging rather than music-making stage the xylophone is an interesting but fairly limited toy so it is useful to choose one that includes other activities as well. For example, several pull-along xylophones have been produced. Mothercare have one mounted on a large plastic lorry called a 'Xylotruck' (£5); Kiddicraft have a 'Musical Fire Engine' which as well as a swivelling xylophone ladder has two bells that ring as it is pulled along and a drum skin mounted on it. The Fisher-Price 'Pull-a-tune Xylophone' plays a tune as it is pulled along and has a colour key so that older children can learn to play simple tunes on it.

Xylophones are also good for encouraging imitative play. Show the child how to bang each key in turn to produce a scale or to run the stick down the whole of the keys. If he can copy these try more complicated things such as seeing if he can copy hitting once, twice or three times on one key or hitting once on each of two different keys.

More Complicated Musical Toys

These toys are a useful and enjoyable way to get a child to engage in a sequence of activities. Because of the various skills involved you will find you need to do rather more teaching than with the simpler musical toys before children can be expected to play constructively with them on their own. They are best used with an adult to help, especially with destructive or heavy-handed children.

The Fisher-Price Music Box Record Player is one of the sturdiest and most widely available. It needs no battery or needle and plays ten different tunes on five strong plastic records. The child has to learn a sequence of four activities. First he has to wind it up, then put a record on the turntable, then put the arm on and finally slide a switch to set it going. Teach him each activity in turn. Some children find the knob stiff and still cannot wind it up even when they can do the rest so you may need to wind it up for the child. The thing is to maintain a balance between keeping his interest and enjoyment in the toy and getting him to learn to do as much as possible for himself. The same sort of strategy applies when showing a child how to work the Matchbox 'Musical Slide'. This has been a big favourite in the Toy Library. Small people ride up a moving staircase as the handle is turned and a tune played. When they get to the top they whizz down the slide. Fisher-Price have also just brought out a musical 'Ferris Wheel' which revolves and plays a tune when wound up and has detachable people who ride in the ferris wheel seats.

Skills taught: FINE MOTOR CO-ORDINATION
SEQUENCING ACTIVITIES
CAUSE AND EFFECT

Fascination Toys

There is a whole 'rag-bag' of toys that are particularly good at getting a child's attention and holding his interest. Most of them are toys that do something visually attractive such as spinning or moving in a particular way. They are especially useful with children who show little interest in toys or do not attend to things for more than a few seconds; or unsociable children who do not usually interact with people or unco-operative children. Particularly with less skilled children, it is often the adult who operates the toy for the child's amusement and can therefore use it as a reward for the child's co-operation.

The following is just a small selection of 'fascination' toys:

Spinning Tops   — especially perspex-topped ones with moving parts inside
(e.g. Novelty toys available from ESA and some toy shops).
Tumbling Toys   — traditional bear or clown who click-clacks down a ladder
(e.g. Tumble Bear by Casden).
Bubble Blowers   — readily available.
Slinkeys   — ESA produce a large size one in plastic.
Kaleidoscopes   — readily available (e.g. ESA).
Wind up Toys   — lots of these available in toy and gift shops. Look out for

	ones with interesting movements such as twirling arms or bobbing head.
Flutterball	– large perspex ball with a rotating butterfly (Playskool): a lovely toy for babies and toddlers but rather fragile.
Leybourne Colour Frames	– three different colours in large light sturdy frames; can be hung up to change the colour of what you see through them.

Skills taught: CONTROL OF ATTENTION
CAUSE AND EFFECT

Pull- and Push-alongs

So many of these are available that just a few we have found especially popular and hard wearing are mentioned here (see also pp. 39-42).

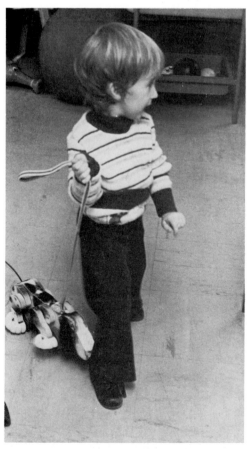

Melody Push Chime (Fisher-Price)	— very sturdy: makes a good noise as it goes round.
Rattle Ball (Fisher-Price)	— perspex ball on frame with small balls that rumble round and make a satisfying noise inside.
Little Snoopy (Fisher-Price)	— an all time favourite: makes a loud click-clack noise as it goes along. Springy tail.
Chatter Telephone (Fisher-Price)	— makes a pleasant clacking sound as it is pulled along and eyes rotate. Can be used as an ordinary toy phone as well.
Clatter Pillar (Kiddicraft)	— another great favourite: visually attractive and intriguing to watch.

These are basically toys you should be able to leave a child to enjoy on his own, with perhaps a little bit of help and demonstration to start with. This does not mean you should never join in: you can often start off imaginative games by asking 'Where are you taking Snoopy? Are you going to give him a drink?'

CHAPTER 5

Toddlers (1-3 Years): Extending the Range of Play

Chapter 4 introduced examples of toys especially suitable for this age (or ability level) and the skills that they can be used to teach. This chapter goes on to describe ways in which different types of play can be encouraged in children who do not develop them spontaneously.

Energetic Play

Early energetic play is often encouraged by social play with an adult. This starts with games like being tossed in the air and jogged on a knee when he is a baby and then develops into catch and chase type games when he can move around and a whole variety of other games such as running at an adult and being swung round. Whereas most children seem to need little encouragement in this area some children who are timid and nervous or lethargic do need more stimulation. Again it takes some handicapped children longer than usual to learn the skills involved in crawling, walking, etc. and it is probably harder work for them so that greater incentives are needed. Remember that nervous or inactive children are often at their most responsive and relaxed as far as energetic play is concerned if it involves an adult rather than a toy.

Generally speaking, the sort of toys you would give to any child are appropriate but bearing certain points in mind. Make sure that baby walkers are heavy and solid and will not tip over easily. The sturdiest traditional wooden ones with bricks inside are fairly expensive but probably the safest from this point of view; look for one that is about the right height for your child. Mother-care have an attractive baby walker in the shape of a bear that can also be sat on and ridden by pushing along with the feet. Some children object to anything new so give him time to get used to the toy being around before trying to persuade him to have a turn: do not force a child on to a toy if he is nervous, and when putting him onto a sit-on toy hold him firmly round his back so he feels supported and do not let go suddenly. Show him how to hold on to the steering wheel or handle and only gradually withdraw your support as he becomes more confident. Many children find it easier to push so that they go backwards rather than forwards to begin with. Do not discourage this unless it persists for a long time as most children will change to forward pushing of their own accord.

If the child is very floppy or is very nervous of sit-on toys you can choose ones that give extra support, such as the traditional rocking horse with an enclosed seat. Another alternative that gives even more support is the Snugglegg by ESA (£11). This is a plastic toy on wheels with a completely enclosed seat in the middle. If the child is happy to sit without support, a whole variety of attractive sit and push-alongs are available. Some tip up easily because of the position of the seat or their general lightness so check them carefully. Many include a lid with a storage chamber which adds interest. A great favourite in the Toy Library is a little blue sit-on milk float that has plastic milk bottles with detachable lids that can be fitted in recesses in the sides. Ones like this are also very useful for encouraging imaginative play and social play with an adult or other children. Pedalling is a skill which many children, but especially poorly co-ordinated children, take a long time to master so one of these sit and push-along with the feet toys is more suitable to start with.

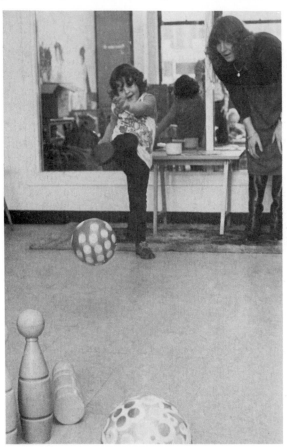

The toys that provide extra support are the safety swing seat by Galt (£4.30), and the rocker type see-saws with enclosed bucket seats (ESA £28; Galt £25.37). As well as toys to sit and ride in there are toys that are useful for encouraging skills like running, jumping and throwing such as a large set of plastic skittles or a set of hoops (Galt Skittles £3.35; Hoops 75p each) or a nursery trampoline (Galt £25.85).

If your child is rather clumsy in his movements play games to give him practice. You can for instance set out several hoops and see if he can step or jump from hoop to hoop. If he appreciates imaginative play this can easily be jumping from island to island. You could also have a narrow band of material or paper as a path or river he has to walk along. Energetic play with an adult is also a very good way of building up social interaction, turn taking and co-operation. For example, when he has learnt to take turns at playing skittles with an adult, introduce another child into the game (easier if it is one who has also learnt to take turns already). If you want to encourage positive inter-action between the children get them to hand the ball to each other and if possible for one to say 'Go!' when it is the other's turn to throw the ball. The illustration shows Peter kicking the ball at the skittles when given the word 'Go' by an adult.

Social and Imitative Play

Social play is not confined to particular kinds of activities or toys. It is some-thing that can be an aspect of most of a child's play as it really consists of any positive or co-operative interaction he has with another person. Even when doing a simple puzzle or stacking some bricks he may look at his mother for approval and encouragement, hand her some bricks or include her with a look in his excitement when the tower falls down. A lot of social play is an integral part of daily activities such as bathing or having tea or going shopping. Before a child has language much of the significance of it for him is transmitted by adult tone of voice, gestures and facial expressions and overall body move-ments, so remember to use these clearly and exaggerate them slightly to get your child's attention and make your meaning clear. Try and dovetail in with the child so that you pick up his glance of expectation or look of interest at something and acknowledge this by showing your own interest or awareness of his expectations. Note how in the illustrations Richard constantly looks at his teacher for encouragement, advice and approval while fitting the wooden men into the Escor boat.

Encouraging Imitative Play

Early imitative play is encouraged by games like clap hands where you first clap your hands and then the child copies. Copying mouth sounds such as lip

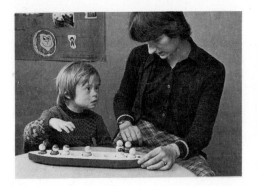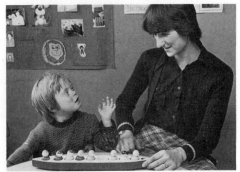

smacking is another form of early imitation. Most children imitate quite spontaneously and frequently but some slow learning children only imitate occasionally or not at all. You may therefore need to make deliberate opportunities to teach him to imitate — either copying something you do with a toy or object ('object orientated' imitation) or where the child copies some sort of body movement ('motor' imitation).

A first step is to make sure that he is attending to the model you are making. Choose something interesting and eye-catching, preferably something you know your child can do of his own accord or that you think he will find easy to learn. The hardest part often is getting them to look at your model so you should call the child's name or choose something noisy like banging on a table. (Sometimes something novel works well but remember they have to be able to do it as well!) If your child is more interested in objects than people you could start by, for example, shaking a bell or squeezing a squeaky hammer as your model for him. Once he has watched your model, prompt him if necessary by taking his hand and guiding him through the activity. This is where it is an advantage to have an activity that is rewarding in itself, although you should always give praise and encouragement as well. You may need to do this several times before he realises that what you want him to do is copy what you have just done.

For children with poor attention or with very poor short-term memory it is useful to have two adults involved so that one of you can make the model whilst the other prompts him to copy it. Sometimes an older brother or sister can be useful here to join in the game but not one near enough in age to be 'in competition'. Some children find 'motor' imitation (copying body movements) harder than 'object' imitation. This is probably because in motor imitation the model disappears as soon as you have finished making it whereas in object imitation the end product (e.g. bricks on a cup) is there to jog the child's memory. It is better to start with two different models the child has to copy such as the squeeze hammer or shake bells so that he learns from the beginning to watch carefully for what model is made. Otherwise there is the danger with one model that he will simply learn that everytime you do something he must clap his hands without really noticing what the thing is that you do. With objects there is also the problem of stopping the child picking them up before you have made your model: keep them out of his reach if necessary and move them towards him only when you want him to make his model. Ideally, to prevent grabbing, it is better to have two sets of objects, one each, but in practice you can manage with one set, although you will probably be better off teaching object imitation at a table where it is easier to control what happens.

The most important thing when you have taught a child to imitate in a teaching session is that this generalises to his everyday play. Generalising from one situation or event to another is something many slow learning children find difficult to do. Encourage it by teaching him to imitate a wide variety of activities in a wide variety of situations. Play games like 'Simple Simon Says' to music and recite nursery rhymes where he can copy your actions. Play games with toys where you do one activity and he does another and you then swop over. I have found with the Matchbox music slide that if I hold a beaker to catch the people as they come down the slide that many children will spontaneously swop over with me and have a go at catching while I operate the slide.

Remember to keep your imitation teaching within the child's abilities. If he has very poor co-ordination, for example, stick to activities he can manage such as knocking over a tower of beakers or hitting a large soft ball suspended on a string.

Activities to Encourage Social Play

No particular type of activity or toy has the monopoly on social play but at the same time it is true that some types of activities and toys are more likely to foster social play than others. Object orientated activities which require the child to concentrate carefully, such as shape and colour matching or doing puzzles, are less likely to develop social play than more open-ended activities, like puppet play or a skittle or ball game, where it is easier for others to be included or to take a turn. At this stage the child is not very aware of the needs or role of other people and play is very much centred around himself (ego-centric). Social play is largely dependent on an adult fitting in with what the child wants to do, and although he will learn to start to take turns with an adult in a game he enjoys, he is unlikely to take turns with other children unless it is carefully engineered. With skittles, for example, hand the ball to one child and keep the other occupied until the first one has had his go. Gather the ball yourself and hand it to the second child, keeping the first occupied. Try and set them to watch each other's throw so they build up an interest in somebody else playing and gradually learn to enjoy taking turns.

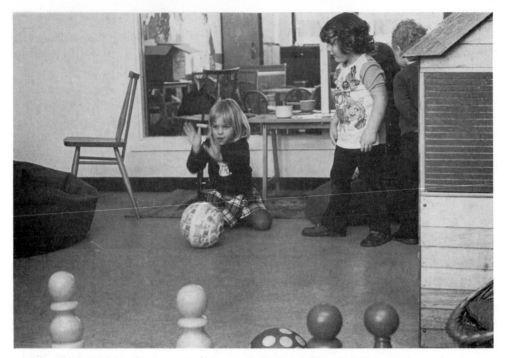

For a child who rarely interacts socially with other children or is unco-operative towards them the nursery rocker type see-saw is ideal because in order to operate it he needs another child. If he enjoys rocking in it place him in it or near it when there is not another child there. It is surprising how often even a very antisocial child will go and find a companion. If he does not do this of his own accord, lead him up to another child and then take them both to the see-saw. He may object until he realises what the point of fetching another child is. This is a particularly good example but you will be able to think of other toys and games where he needs to co-operate with an adult or child in order to get enjoyment.

Imaginative Play

Imaginative play usually starts around one to one-and-a-half years with delayed imitation of things he has seen, like brushing his hair, and play with largish models of familiar household objects such as teasets. He will also push a car along making appropriate 'brrm-brrm' noises. At about two years imaginative play such as feeding and nursing dolls starts to expand rapidly and is no longer purely imitative but is also inventive. Once a child begins to show signs of realising that miniature toys like model farm animals or dolls' house furniture are *representations* of things in the real world, he is ready to enjoy imaginative play. Whereas a teaset will have been used more like nesting beakers before, simply as objects to line up or stack, he will now pretend to drink from the cup or pour a cup of tea or hand you a cup of tea. Lots of teasets, cooking sets, pastry sets and cleaning sets are available: Galt and ESA both have a good selection of these. Most are plastic but Galt have a set of saucepans in shiny metal which children find particularly attractive and satisfying to play with. Fisher-Price have just brought out a kitchen set which has a two ring cooker top with controls and accompanying utensils and tea set. In our Toy Library children of both sexes have been equally fascinated by our model cooker and saucepans so do not just think of these as being toys for girls. As well as promoting imaginative play these sort of toys are useful for encouraging social play.

For children who are slow to develop imaginative play, toys that are interesting in their own right are preferable, as some like the Fisher-Price nursery set are only really of interest to the child when he knows roughly what the pieces are, and before this time are likely to be given a cursory examination and cast away. Many children find a model hoover or carpet sweeper interesting to use in the way they would any push- or pull-along before they necessarily appreciate what it represents. Similarly, some find the Escor wooden roundabout interesting and like taking the men in and out before they give any indication of 'knowing' what the models are. Try to foster imaginative play by walking the model men along and jumping them into their seats. Apart from the Escor range there are a whole host of plastic cars, boats, and so on, complete with their own drivers that can form the basis of exciting and boisterous chases. However, toys where small parts are involved are obviously vulnerable to breakage if treated inappropriately. If you are not sure how your child will play with one of these start with a simple robust toy such as a play family mini bus or fire engine (both Fisher-Price) and see how he treats it. Does he show signs of appreciating that the model figures are 'people' or does he simply bang the toy about and treat the people like pegs?

Some children, even when they show some awareness that these things are models, are poor at playing with them imaginatively. The weeble playground, for example, has a set of swings, a slide and a roundabout but needs all these activities demonstrated before many children appreciate what can be done. Some children lose concentration very quickly and rarely carry out a structured activity. To encourage more persistence you can join in the whole activity — for example, make a big game of you both jumping men up to the slide in turn and then jumping them up the steps. Then let them slide down into a container or let them fall down the table to the floor. Similarly with the swings make a big event of jumping one of the weebles on to the swing and saying 'Push' when you are going to push it. Prompt the child if necessary, but often if you do this with the first weeble he will copy with the second one.

We have found the Palitoy Tree House very successful as a first dolls' house for children of both sexes. With its spring-up opening action, wind up and down lift, brightly coloured parts and additions like a swing and kennel, it appeals to children who may not yet be ready to get a lot of play out of a more conventional type of dolls' house and at £12 is pretty good value for money. As with the weebles playground, demonstrate the various activities that are possible and then encourage the child to do them himself.

Another type of toy that is useful for both imaginative and imitative play is the hand puppet. Large versions of these in the shape of Kermit and many other popular characters are available. Demonstrate to your child how Kermit can sleep, wave, jump, etc. and either get him to copy Kermit or get him to do similar things with Kermit himself. Do not forget that although speech often seems to play a large role in imaginative play, you can have children who show by their use of toys quite a high level of imaginative play despite the fact that they are not yet talking. In fact, one of the first and most popular toys to be recognised as a model is the toy telephone (although the real one always seems to be of greater interest!) Play with the child and encourage him to pretend to listen and 'speak' on the phone even if he is not yet using words.

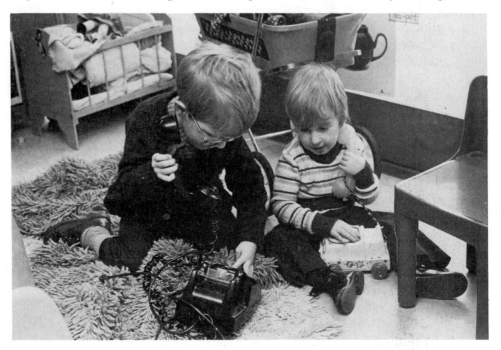

Language Development

Like social play, language play is not confined to particular activities and toys, but again certain types of activities and toys are more likely to enhance it. First it is useful to divide language into two areas: *receptive*, that is the language the child hears and understands; and *expressive*, which is the language the child speaks. Most children learn to understand language before they can speak it and this is of course necessary if what they are going to say is to be meaningful and appropriate. If, for example, a child could say the word 'cup' but had no idea what a cup was, he would not use this word to indicate that he had seen a cup or wanted a cup but would just come out with it at random times. In this case he would not have learnt that language is about *communicating* something to somebody else or at least labelling and categorising something for himself.

To understand what words mean and what communication is, a child needs experience in all areas of development. He needs to know what objects are, he needs to know what putting 'in' and taking 'out' is, what running, jumping and walking are. He also needs to know what effect his 'communication' has on other people. He will gradually learn from babyhood that if he looks at something an adult may follow his gaze and share his point of interest. Later he learns to point or gesture and to make noises to indicate his interests and needs. So that by the time he comes to speaking he has already learnt quite a lot about what it is to communicate.

It is tempting to get a young child, particularly if he is behind and you are anxious about his progress, to speak as soon and as much as possible. Although in the long run you obviously want him to speak, it is more important that you first teach him to understand and not just to talk like a parrot. It is tempting to teach young children lots of nursery rhymes and such like and, whereas this does not really matter with a child who is developing a good understanding of language, with a child who is slow to develop this, the rhymes will be largely meaningless and will not be teaching him to communicate.

Toys and Activities for Encouraging Language Play

Many of the toys and activities mentioned already will be useful for helping both receptive and expressive language. Toys like the Musical Slide (Matchbox) and the Tree House (Palitoy), the weeble playground and the Escor Roundabout are all useful for encouraging a wide range of language skills.

Others that can be added to the list are:

Play Family Fun Jet, Airport, House, Garage — all Fisher-Price;
Family Ferry, Family Camper — Matchbox;
Joggle Train — Palitoy;
Noah's Chuckle Ark, Carousel — both Corgi.

All these are good for encouraging action as well as labelling words.

Pictures are useful and need to be as clear and uncluttered as possible to begin with. Available from ESA are 'Talking Picture' — a set of twelve very large photographs of everyday objects such as a spoon and a telephone; 'First Words' cards (105 photographs) which are also very popular; and Giant Picture

Lotto, in use in the accompanying illustration.

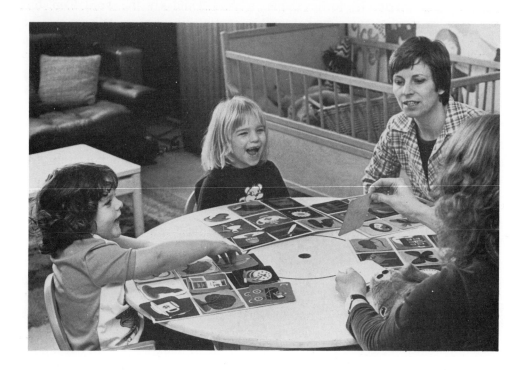

Table 5.1: Early Insets and Puzzles for Encouraging Language

Name	Comment	Manufacturer or Supplier
See inside Jigsaws Shops Cars Farm	Long trays with 5 or 6 lift out pieces such as the cars and lorries on the Traffic tray.	Galt £3 each
Stand up Jigsaws Farm 200	14 animals that lift out and stand up — each one nice and clear.	Galt £3 each
Abbatt Inset Puzzles Garden House Kitchen Cupboards	'See inside' type insets. Lift out the pieces such as the cupboard doors and see what is inside.	ESA £2.95 each
Picture Trays Country Traffic	Large trays with several large clear lift out pieces.	ESA £5.95
Meal Time Jigsaws	Clear photographic prints mounted on wood. Action in each picture. Several pieces that can be lifted out.	Four to Eight £3.65 each

Table 5.1: Continued

Name	Comment	Manufacturer or Supplier
Everyday Object Pictures Dustpan and Brush Telephone Teapot and Cups Cat, etc.	Photographic Print Puzzles with between 2 and 14 pieces. Very clear and attractive to children.	Four to Eight £3.65 each
Inset Puzzles Tea Time Circus	Lovely jigsaws in 3D. Pieces can be taken out and stood up. Good for action words as well as labelling.	Susan Wynter £2.50 each
Tray Jigsaws Clothes Pots n' Pans	Pieces all fit in a frame. Lots of pictures on a tray around one theme.	Susan Wynter £2 each
Transport Insets Bus Road Traffic Train	'See inside' type insets. Bright clear pictures are more complicated than any of the previous puzzles. Useful for expanding parts of speech.	E.J. Arnold
Raised Insets Puzzles Breakfast Washing	Easy to lift out pieces — excellent for encouraging language.	John Adam's Toys

Table 5.2: Early Picture Books

Name	Comment	Publisher or Supplier
Things I see e.g. Traffic, Animals, etc.	Clearly printed pictures on very thick board that is hard to rip.	Galt 60p each

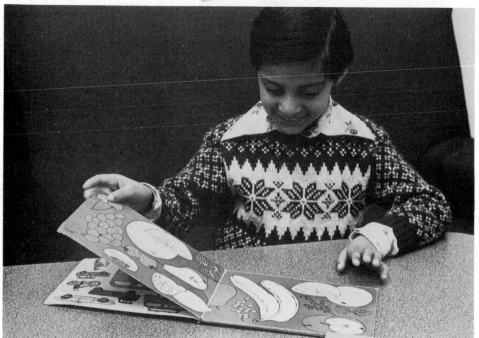

Baby's First Book Picture Book ABC Book	All have clear pictures of objects.	Ladybird
About the House Book	Clear pictures of household objects. Several related objects to a page.	Philip and Tacey

Table 5.2: Continued

Name	Comment	Publisher or Supplier

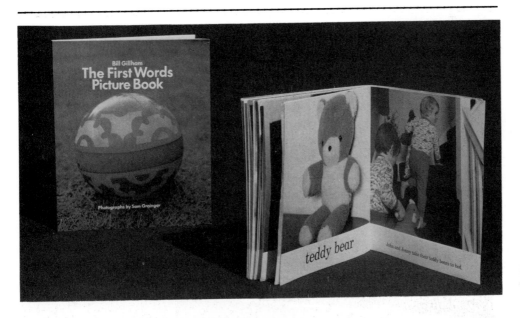

Name	Comment	Publisher or Supplier
First Words Picture Book	Attractive coloured photographs with simple text covering the 15 'topics' that children talk about first (see illustration).	Methuen Bill Gillham
Talkabouts The Home The Garden Shopping	Most topics relevant to a child's everyday life.	Ladybird
First Picture 1 First Picture 2 Learn to Look 1 Learn to Look 2	Printed on heavy card. Suggestions and ideas for teaching with each book.	Barnaby Books (C. Cunningham & D. Jeffree) LDA, Wisbech
First Sentences Cards	Sets of line drawings with 2-word sentences to make up into books (see illustration).	LDA, Wisbech (Bill Gillham & Paul Livock)

Finally, a couple of unusual toys that are specifically centered around language. First, the Fisher-Price Pocket Camera. This is about the size of an instamatic camera and shows 27 slides of a trip to the zoo. For those children who like active or mechanical type toys but will rarely sit down and play with puzzles or look at pictures in books, it is an attractive alternative to focus attention while you talk about what is going on. Another unusual toy is the Mattel Animal Clock (illustrated). A large arrow is pointed to one of the pictures of an animal and when the cord at the side is pulled an amazing American accent says things like 'Do you hear the fr-o-o--g (frog)?', followed by the appropriate animal noise.

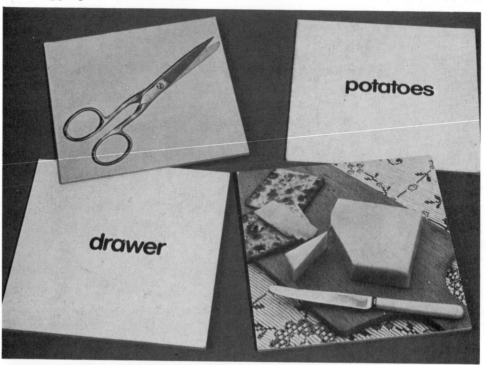

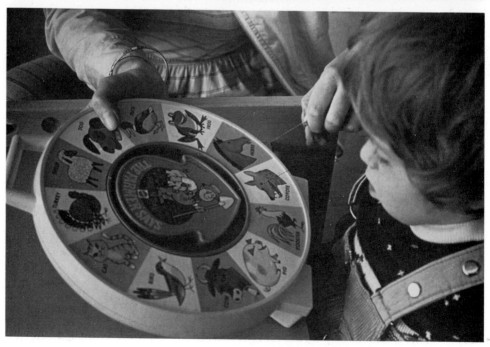

Finding Out What He Understands

It is useful to start by trying to establish how much language your child already understands.

(1) Does he turn to his name?
(2) Does he seem to respond to words like dinner, Daddy, car, etc.?
(3) Does he react to yes and no?
(4) Does he understand simple phrases like 'put it down', 'come here' or 'tea's ready'?
(5) Could he go and fetch you something from another room?
(6) Could he answer a question even if by pointing or gesture, e.g. 'Do you want milk or orange?'
(7) Does he understand what words like 'in', 'on', and 'out' mean?
(8) Could he carry out a complicated instruction, e.g. 'Go and get your brown shoes and put them under the chair'?

When trying to find out how much the child understands, be careful not to give him clues by your gestures and eye gaze. Even without realising it you often glance, for example, at the light switch before telling him to switch it on. You also tend to ask the child to do the same things as part of a routine so when you get your bag out to go shopping you might tell him to fetch his coat; but you do not know if he has really understood what you have *said* or is just inferring from the situation that you are going shopping. Try asking him to fetch his coat without making any preparations for going out and at a time you do not usually go and see how he responds. A more systematic way of assessing his receptive language or comprehension is to lay out several familiar objects and ask him to point or hand you certain ones. If he is not able to pick out the right one at first you can start with just two dissimilar but familiar objects, e.g. a cup and a teddy, and say something like 'Can I have the cup? Will you give me the cup?' and at the same time point to it and hold your hand out expectantly. Prompt him if he does not pick it up himself. Do this until he can pick up both objects correctly and then introduce more objects or play find games where he has to look for the named object in a cardboard box. You can also try this with the ESA Giant Snap Cards or the First Words Picture Cards, mentioned earlier. These are also good for early naming games, 'Oo, what's this?', and if there is no reply, 'I think it's TEDDY', etc. Once your child knows what various common objects are called, do not push him to label them all the time just for the sake of it to show off his knowledge to other people as this is not teaching the child about 'communication' and he may well start refusing to talk on these occasions.

When he knows what some everyday objects are, even if he is not yet saying the words himself, encourage him to understand verbs or action words like 'go', 'stop', 'come', and later prepositions like 'in', 'on', and 'under'. Toys like the weebles playground and the matchbox musical slide are ideal for introducing these. Active games are another way of encouraging understanding and use of action words. You can say 'Jump' or 'Run' or 'Kick' as you do the activity. '*Up* we go! Who can jump *up*?', and so on (see illustration).

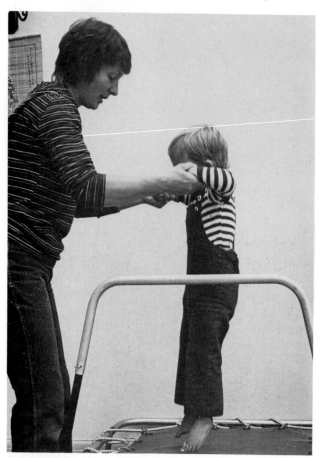

To help expand your child's receptive language you can play games where he has to follow a phrase or short sentence. For example, 'Put Kermit in the box', 'Sit teddy on the chair.' At first he will probably pick out key words like teddy and chair but later you can play games where he has to put teddy on, under, in front of or behind the chair so he learns these sort of words as well. The Susan Wynter tea-time puzzle with its stand up pieces is ideal for this sort of language play. You can ask questions like 'Can you put the girl on the chair?' 'Can you put the cat under the table?', and so on.

When the child is saying 20 or more words, if he is not spontaneously starting to put words together, try to encourage this through language play. For example, with the puppet game, encourage the child to say 'Kermit's sleeping', 'Kermit's waving', etc. At first you may have to do this in two stages. When he has said 'sleeping', you ask 'Who's sleeping?' and supply the answer 'Kermit' for him then to say 'Kermit's sleeping'. It is easier to do this with two words he already knows, so if he is saying some kind of action word like 'gone' or 'down', couple it with a labelling word like 'teddy' or 'cup' and incorporate it in a game of 'teddy's gone!', 'cup's gone!' as you drop them into a box.

If a child can understand quite a lot of what you say but is not saying a lot himself, another useful technique is forced choice questions. In this case you ask him a question like 'Do you want pop or milk?' and wait for his answer. The advantage of this is that he does not have to think of the correct word himself: he just has to choose it from the two words you present him with. You can also use this technique to encourage him to use adjectives and adverbs (descriptive words). 'Do you want a green sweet or a red sweet?'

This is in fact part of a game we play with our language group. Smarties and other small objects are hidden in some Tupperware click together bricks, and each child can choose which box he wants to open by saying either 'blue box' or 'red box'. Another popular game is giving each child a choice of what they want Kermit to do. 'Do you want Kermit to run quickly or run slowly?'

To summarise here are a few general guidelines:

(1) Remember that many handicapped children are poor at switching attention so make sure he is listening to you and is not still absorbed in some other activity.
(2) Do not swamp him with language. Keep sentences short and clear and stress the words you want him to notice, e.g. 'Put teddy DOWN' or 'Yes, it's a TELEPHONE'.
(3) If you are trying to find out how much spoken language he understands make sure that you are not giving him clues through gesture and the situation.
(4) At other times help his understanding of language by accompanying your words by gestures but remember to fade these out gradually if you can.
(5) If you are using insets and jigsaws primarily to encourage language, concentrate on talking about the pictures and the pieces rather than teaching him to fit them in. The next section suggests how to get the best use from them and gives further examples.

Insets and Jigsaws

Insets usually consist of a board or tray with several pieces that can be taken out; some like the Galt See Inside Insets and the ESA Inset Puzzles have knobs on the pieces to make it easier to take them in and out. Others like the ESA picture trays and the Galt stand up puzzles have raised pieces that are thicker than the board. In some instances the pieces are an integral part of an all over picture such as a traffic scene or a farm scene whereas in others, like the Galt stand up farm, the pieces which are all animals fit into a plain green background.

Probably the most popular insets for starting with in our Toy Library are the Galt See Inside insets and stand up farm puzzles and the ESA picture trays. These all have relatively large clear pictures which are of interest to most children. At this stage a child is really being given a shape matching task, that is, he has to match the 'car' shaped piece to a 'car' shaped inset on the board. The next step on from this is a cross between an inset and a jigsaw. There is still a background that the pieces fit into but instead of fitting separately the pieces fit together to form a picture of an object. At this stage the child can match by shape and picture. Four to Eight have a very realistic set of object pictures graded in difficulty from two to 14 pieces that are ideal as an introduction to this sort of puzzle. Both ESA and Galt have a good range of these tray type jigsaws. They all generally have pieces that do not interlock but 'slide fit' into place so the child can concentrate on matching up the picture without also being involved in the difficult and easily discouraging task of fitting interlocking pieces together.

As a first introduction to interlocking puzzles the ESA colour picture puzzles are a good step. These consist of a separate picture each being constructed of two pieces that interlock along one side. The next step on from there is probably the simplest of the Giant Floor Jigsaws which have 15-25 pieces. Four to Eight produce an attractive Circus and Noah's Ark, Galt have a very clearly printed Fruit and Vegetable one (available from E.J. Arnold) and Candor have a selection of three delightful pictures. These are mounted on wood so that the pieces are easy to handle and will not buckle and break when brute force rather than skill is used to try and fit them together.

Teaching Techniques

With the early insets present them to the child and talk about the pictures as suggested in the Language section. Demonstrate taking the pieces out or tipping them out for children who would find taking them out difficult. If you find he has difficulty grasping the knobs or raised pieces larger knobs can be fitted — both small size wooden or plastic cupboard knobs and golf tees make good ones. With the golf tees push the tapered end through the existing hole or drill a larger hole if necessary. Trim off the excess and melt the tee at the back of the puzzle to fix it securely in place. Alternatively, simple insets with extra large knobs known as Giant Knob Puzzles are available from Globe Education and some shops.

It is better to have the child sitting at a table or kneeling at a lower surface so he has both hands free and has the puzzle directly in front of him. When children play with them on the floor they are often supporting themselves with one hand or sitting in a position where they have to reach to pull the pieces out.

Putting the pieces back is quite a different skill which requires complex shape matching and good eye–hand co-ordination. Many children make some haphazard attempts to put the pieces back in but rapidly give up because of their lack of success. Make the task easier for the child by breaking it down into steps and structuring it for him. There are a variety of ways in which you can do this. You could, for example, with the empty Galt traffic inset, just present him with one car in the correct orientation and point to the correct slot for him to put it in and then if necessary take his hand and guide him through the action of fitting the car in. Alternatively, you could place the car just below or even half in the correct slot and just prompt him to push it right in. This is a good technique with children who give up very easily or are difficult to prompt.

The child is faced with the problem of learning both a matching and a fitting task. At first, therefore, do the matching for him so he can concentrate on the fitting. When you know he can fit the pieces in easily hand him one and see what he does. If he starts to go towards the wrong slot say 'no' and see if he will correct himself. You can, of course, let the child try and fit the piece in by trial and error until he comes to the right slot but this tends to lead to frustration for the child and may mean that he will carry on with this method for some time and not learn to search for the correct slot. Some children do not scan the board first but just try and fit the piece into the first slot they see. In this case prompt the child by pointing your finger all round the board to encourage him to scan the whole board first. Another method is to hold the piece in turn by each slot and get the child to signal with your 'yes' or 'no' as to whether it is the correct one. Other children are haphazard in their approach: they grab a number of pieces in each hand and hopefully ram them at the board. Teach the child to pick up only one piece at a time. You can get him into the habit of this by only presenting him with one piece and keeping the rest out of his way (sit on them if necessary!). Gradually introduce the rest at a distance and then all the pieces together first pointing out one particular piece for him to pick up.

Once the child can do simple insets it is time to move on to insets where he has to fit the pieces together to make a picture or object. These insets vary in how much help they give the child. Language can be used to guide his performance and help him pay attention to new cues, that is the picture rather than just the shape. With the Abbatt Snowman, for example, you might guide the child by saying:

'Find his hat';
'Yes, that's his hat';
'Try it at the top';

'Turn it round';
'Find her other leg';
'Where's her other leg?';
'Oo, I think that's the snowman's scarf';
'Where will his scarf go?';
'Round his neck, yes that's right'.

This is a very useful teaching technique with children who have a fair understanding of language and teaches them to label and identify pieces of puzzle and look out for the logical or likely place for such a part to go (i.e. the child making use of ideas like legs go at the bottom of bodies and heads go at the top of bodies). The same technique can be extended to doing simple interlocking puzzles like the Giant Floor Puzzles. In this case it is not always possible to label each piece so teach him to find 'another stripey piece', 'another red piece', etc. Some children find it a help to put all the straight edged pieces together first, so help them to look out for and identify these pieces.

One problem with doing a lot of insets is that a child gets used to being able to slide two pieces together and sometimes tries to do the same unsuccessfully with interlocking type puzzle pieces. The two piece colour picture puzzles are useful for teaching a child how to put interlocking pieces together. Demonstrate to him that you have to lift one piece up and fit it onto the next piece. These two piece puzzles are also ideal for teaching him to match pieces by picture and not shape. Start by having out, say, two halves of car and one half of shoe. Have one half of car and one half of shoe and see if he can pick the correct half. If necessary help him by pointing or guiding his hand to the correct piece. When he can do this give him four halves muddled up and see if he can still do it. Try out all the various combinations of pictures and gradually increase the number of pieces you give him to match up until he can cope with all eighteen halves out at once.

CHAPTER 6

Pre-school and Nursery (3-5 Years)

Skills to Develop

(1)   Understanding most of what is said to him.
(2)   Talking in complete sentences and using all parts of speech.
(3)   Good motor skills including running, jumping and pedalling a bike.
(4)   Naming colours and counting out four or five objects accurately.
(5)   Planning and carrying out elaborate constructive play such as building a Lego model.
(6)   Engaging in long sequences of imaginative and role play.
(7)   Drawing a man.
(8)   Enjoying listening to stories.
(9)   Learning to follow simple rules in playing games (e.g. Snap and Picture Lotto).
(10) Starting to play sociably with other children.
(11) Dressing and undressing.

By the time a child has developed most of the skills listed at the beginning of Chapter 4, he will be ready to generate a lot of his own learning, especially in areas like imaginative and constructive play. Whilst formal skills such as counting, colour naming and picture matching become appropriate at this stage, it is important to encourage all forms of play as they all add to a child's global understanding of concepts like number and size. It is also important in encouraging these sorts of skills more systematically and directly, to keep the activities at an enjoyable 'fun' level for the child. As ever there are wide variations in children's personalities and whereas one child seems positively to enoy a 'work' session, another child will be totally unco-operative and more entertaining means of teaching him will have to be found.

Number Play

Teaching numbers to a handicapped child is no different in principle from teaching them to any child. It may be that they are slower or less likely to pick it up for themselves and may need more help or practice with the various stages.

Many children learn to count by rote. In other words they can say 'one, two, three, four, five, etc.' but this is not the same as being able to count out a number of objects accurately which is what understanding number really involves. A young child will often start counting out objects and yet have a completely different number of objects to the number he is saying. As with language, rather than going straight for *saying* numbers, we need to go for the concepts or understanding of number that underlie counting. These can be built up in a variety of ways.

First, try games to make the child aware of having 'one' as opposed to 'two' objects. If you have been handing him one weeble at a time for the slide you could hold out two weebles asking him, 'Would you like *two* weebles?' or when playing a fitting game you could hand him two pegs or ask him to give you two pegs. You can reinforce this through a variety of situations. Does he want one or two biscuits? How many boots has he got? Try and get him to pick two things that are the same out of a group of three. You could, for example, put out three Giant Snap cards, two with pictures of a teddy and one with a picture of a shoe, and ask for the two teddies. This will help teach him that numbers consist of groups of things that are the same. To start with this can be kept at a simple and concrete level, but later he will also learn that a number could consist of a group of things called animals as opposed to flowers. In this instance he is learning that things go into categories according to certain features they share such as legs and eyes as opposed to petals, etc.

Once children get beyond the numbers one and two, part of the difficulty they encounter is a spatial one of not remembering where they have started counting from so they often count one object twice, or completely miss one out or, as mentioned before, get their spoken counting out of time with their finger pointing. To help with all these problems, you start by getting the child to take from you or hand to you each object as he counts it. Alternatively you could encourage him to play a game of dropping the objects into a tin or box as he counts them. If you are handing the child the objects, make him wait until you are putting each object in his hand to count it. Keep this going at quite a fast speed as even with counting up to three young children quickly forget where they have got to. By doing this you will teach him to say a number as he handles each object. Next you can try putting three or four objects or pictures on the floor. Have them in a straight line far enough apart for each object to be distinctly separate but not so far apart that he does not even notice the ones at the end. It is easier if you have them in a straight line as the child is then less likely to become confused about which objects he has counted. Start counting at one end, and try to get him to the stage where he just needs to point to each object as he says the number. When he can do this you can put the objects in a group to see if he can remember where he started counting from. A useful game for teaching a child to look for like objects and to count up to three or four is 'Lost and Found' by Kiddicraft where he has to collect three baby animals to match the mother animal.

This learning can be reinforced with informal games and activities. He could count how many red, blue, etc. balloons you blow up or help count out how many cups are needed for tea or how many milk bottles are to go by the door. Many of the Escor, Fisher-Price and Matchbox type toys are ideal for number play. How many people are upstairs? How many are in the car? and so on.

There is a lot involved in learning to count accurately: it is not necessary to make a child stay at the level of two or three objects until he is consistently right before going on to introducing four or more.

Useful Number Games and Puzzles

When he has reached this stage a start can be made with some early number games. One of the best is 'Ladybird, Ladybird' by Orchard Toys. This has cards with up to six large spots on them and on the reverse side a leaf with nought to four ladybirds on it. The cards are laid out spot-side up and a dice thrown. You then pick up a corresponding card and turn it over to see how many ladybirds you have. The winner is the one who collects the most lady-birds. With help this is a reasonably straightforward game for children and involves them in a lot of simple counting. A problem with most of these games is that the dice is really too small for children who still need to count by putting their finger on each dot. It is possible to buy some very large dice from specialist games shops and from Galt and occasionally elsewhere. But it is not too difficult to make one by painting dots carefully on to a plain wooden brick.

Further games that involve numbers one to five are the Galt Number and Sets Lotto and Count and Match Lotto.

Various number type puzzles exist where the child has to match the picture of the object to the correct number of dots or the correct printed number. Some of these go up to ten or even 20, but start by giving the child just the first two or three numbers and only introduce more when he can do these. At this stage always give the child dots or objects (it does not matter if there are printed numerals as well) to match the objects to as knowing which printed numeral stands for what actual number (quantity) is yet another thing the child has to learn. Watch to see if he is actually matching by number – you will probably need to demonstrate this at first – as some children are very good at matching the shapes of the pieces. If he is doing this help him to count the objects and the dots in order to find the matching pieces. Galt produce quite an attractive game called 'Count to 20'. The child has to count the apples on each tree, then find a base piece with the same number of apples.

An unusual toy which is surprisingly popular with children is 'One Dozen

Eggs' by Palitoy. This comprises a life size blue plastic eggbox with a dozen plastic eggs. Each egg consists of two halves which are fitted together by means of pegs in one half being pushed into holes in the other half. Each egg has a differing number of pegs and holes (plus printed numeral) between one and twelve. As with the puzzle type toys you can start by just giving the child the eggs with the first two or three numbers and gradually increase them as he learns to count.

An enjoyable game by Galt that goes up to ten is 'Number Me'; it can be played with either dots or printed numerals. If it not necessary to teach a child printed numerals at this stage but if he seems to be recognising them in games where both dots and numerals are given you could gradually introduce them. The Mothercare clock with large plastic numerals that fit into the clock face is useful for familiarising children with written numbers.

Complex Size, Shape and Colour Matching

A child learns matching skills informally with many of the toys he plays with. For example, sorting out two different size model people for their appropriate toys, or putting the right colour plastic cups in the right colour saucers or choosing the correct pieces of plastic railway to fit together, all involve these skills. But some children learn less in this incidental way than others and need more planned and structured help. There are two ways of doing this. One is to take every opportunity that arises during everyday activities to help develop these skills; so, for example, if a child starts playing with saucepans or tins of food he could be helped to grade and line them up by size or height; or he could be given spoons of various sizes to sort out into the cutlery drawer.

Another way is to provide toys or objects specifically designed to encourage these sorts of skills, although he will still have to be taught how to use them. Ideally a combination of both methods should be used.

There are a lot of board type activities but not so many interesting action toys to teach matching, which is a pity as it is often the children who are least interested in the board games who need the most help. The following four toys all provide a useful bridge between simple and complex matching skills and provide enjoyable practice.

The Palitoy Shape School is an attractive toy with a colourful classroom, swings and roundabouts and a school bus. Each person can only be fitted into the appropriate shaped space by one of the desks. It is a useful toy to introduce to children who like imaginative play but dislike straightforward shape matching toys.

Another interesting toy is the 'Keys of Learning', also by Palitoy. In this case the correct coloured key has to be inserted into each keyhole to raise the appropriate colour shape.

A toy we have found very popular is the Kiddicraft Posting Pagoda, which involves both colour and shape matching. Twelve different shapes can be posted through the doors and roofs of the six-sided house and the six roofs are also fitted on according to shape and colour. The doors are all different colours and can be opened by the matching coloured keys.

Finally, a delightful model toy is 'Mr Postman' by Palitoy. In this case an automatic sorting office loads coloured letters on to a mail van and the letters can only be delivered to the matching colour home.

Teaching Techniques

If a child does not start fitting the correct people into the correct slots in the Shape School, it may be because he has not realised that a shape matching task is involved. It is necessary to get him to pick each person up and turn it over so he can look and see what shape it is and which hole it will fit in. With the two toys involving keys (Keys of Learning and Posting Pagoda) getting the keys into the locks can be quite fiddly and as they are made of plastic they snap if forced. To avoid this it may be necessary to guide the child's hand to fit the keys in and turn them appropriately. With the 'Keys of Learning' you may have to point out what it is he needs to match as the coloured shape is on the top of the box and the corresponding keyhole is directly below on the side of the box.

With the Posting Pagoda you may need to teach the child several steps. Start with the shapes in the house, the roofs on and the doors locked. Hand him one colour key and show him how to turn the box round until he finds the same colour door. Then show him how to insert the key and turn it so he can open the door and take the shapes out. If you are planning to repeat this sequence it is also useful to get him to relock the door afterwards. You can either get him to remove the roof at the same time or remove all the roofs after he has removed all the shapes.

When he has all the shapes, show him how to sort them into colour groups and then to choose one group. Now remind him how to turn the house round until he finds the matching colour door plus roof to post the shapes through. Finally, get him to use the same tactics to fit all the roofs on and then you are back at the beginning of the sequence again. Obviously this is a flexible toy that can be played with in a variety of ways and sequences. The point to teaching one particular sequence is to ensure that he tackles all the skills involved and carries out a complete task from beginning to end rather than just shuffling the shapes rather aimlessly through any open door. Once he can play with it competently you can leave him to experiment as he wishes.

Just to give an example of the diverse ways in which many toys can be used, we have found the Pagoda a useful toy for work with a language group. In the accompanying illustration you can see the sequence described being followed. Each child is asked in turn to choose a colour key by name. When we started, to make it easier, the children were presented with just two keys and given a forced choice question such as 'Do you want a red or a blue key?', but now some of them can name spontaneously the colour key they want. They then have to say what they want to do with the key before the pagoda is passed over to them. On this occasion we are encouraging two word combinations such as 'open door' followed by others such as 'shapes out' and 'close door'. It is interesting to see how a matching type toy like this can also be used to develop entirely different areas of skill and underlines the need to be flexible in our approach to toys and the sort of expectations we have about what they will do. It also shows the vital role of adult intervention and teaching in expanding the use of a toy.

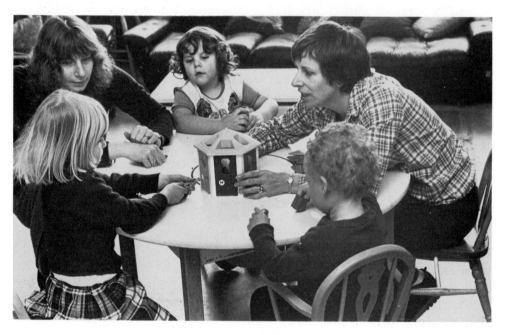

Easy Board Games

Some of these are a good introduction to games with formal rules in general and are very simple and straightforward to play.

Early Birds and Bumble Bee by Kiddicraft, Rainbow Game and Hickory Dickory Dock by Orchard Toys and the Dick Bruna colour Lotto are all interesting games for encouraging colour matching. In Hickory Dickory Dock the child has a large coloured cardboard clock and has to find all the matching colour mice to put on the base of the clock. He then takes turns to throw the special dice which has a picture of a mouse on most sides and a line on a few. If he throws a mouse he can move one of the mice on to the first space on the clock. The winner is the first person to have filled his clock up.

Early Birds and Bumble Bee both involve the child throwing a coloured dice and in one case choosing a piece of the same colour and in the other moving his piece on to an area of the same colour. With the Dick Bruna Lotto the child throws a coloured dice and chooses the appropriate coloured balloon and then fits it on the same colour balloon on his lotto card.

With these early games there is a lot to teach the child. He has to learn to take turns and, probably, needs to develop some idea of what 'winning' is if his interest is to be held by the game. With each game he has to learn the specific routine and conventions peculiar to it. In Hickory Dickory Dock, for example, you may first have to teach him to sort out all the colour mice matching the clock and then where to place them. He may have to be shown how to use a dice for the first time in his life, which involves coming to learn that some symbol or configuration on the dice indicates what he can do. He also has to learn not to move pieces around between his turns and only to move them in a prescribed manner at these times. And he has to develop some idea of what the goal of the game is (i.e. to move all his mice on to the clock) and to appreciate that it will take several goes to reach this goal.

Considering how much is involved it is surprising how children 'catch on' to what is required; but there are many occasions when the game does not seem to get off the ground. Part of the problem is that until you have persuaded the child to go through the game a few times he may not see the point of it or get much enjoyment from it. You can solve this partly by choosing visually attractive games like Hickory Dickory Dock and imparting as much enthusiasm and excitement as you can into the game.

Adult: Oo! It's a mouse! (As child throws dice.)
Let's jump one of your mice onto the clock. (Demonstrates jumping mouse on to clock and returns it quietly to base.)
Do you want to do it? Do you want to jump him into the clock? (Says this whilst pointing to the cardboard mouse.)
(If no response from child . . .)
Shall I put him back on for you?
(If response . . .)
That's it, now it's my go, I wonder if I'm going to get a mouse? etc.

Remember that all these games require the child to learn a lot of new skills, some of which are quite complex and difficult. Many children find moving a counter or piece a specific number of spaces a very hard thing to learn. It is therefore a good idea to play a new game through by yourself or with another adult or older child before introducing it, as this will give you time to work out all the steps involved and to think of effective and interesting ways of teaching.

Notice how in the outline conversation for Hickory Dickory Dock that the adult does not force the child to put the mouse on, but gives him a let out by offering to do it, thus avoiding a possible confrontation situation at a point where the child is not yet very enthusiastic about the game. This is a situation that can often arise when showing a child a new toy and requires the adult to judge whether it is better to prompt him to do the activity or just to ignore his refusal. Part of this decision is based on whether it is a genuine refusal or a question of him not really knowing what to do. If the latter case you will obviously need to give him more help and guidance, whereas in the former case, where you suspect he *could* carry out the activity, you need to increase his willingness and motivation to carry it out or accept that he is not interested and move on to something else.

Complex Board Games

Galt, E.J. Arnold, Philip and Tacey and Four to Eight all have a number of board games that are specifically designed to help with colour, shape and size matching. Most of them would be easier to introduce after a child has had experience of some of the simpler games as they tend to involve more steps and to take longer to play before the goal is reached. As with the earlier games, it is possible to simplify them if a child is encountering difficulty and therefore losing interest. Going back to Hickory Dickory Dock for a moment, this has blank lines on some sides of the dice which in fact indicate that the child should remove a mouse, but for children who get bored quickly and need a short game, it is useful simply to let this indicate that they cannot put a mouse on. The problem then, of course, is that you may have difficulty later on in instituting the full rules, particularly when there are other children joining in who have played before! Modify the rules only where it seems necessary to keep the child involved in the game. We find with 'Build a House' (Galt), for example, that the game takes a long time to finish off and that younger children can get restless so at this point we allow them up to three throws of the dice each to speed things up.

Games

Having already discussed games under the auspices of shape, size and colour matching, this seems a good point at which to introduce some more general games and consider what the child needs to learn and is likely to learn in the process of playing them.

Both Orchard toys and Kiddicraft produce a number of good basic games. Two of the easiest to play are 'What time is it, Mr Wolf?' and 'Insey Winsey Spider'. Mr Wolf is a ghoulish game that many children seem to delight in and many parents seem to tire of quickly because of the incessant demand to play it. In this game one person is Mr Wolf and the others ask in turn, 'What time is it, Mr Wolf?', as in the traditional game. Mr Wolf then spins the dial on his clock. If it lands in the red area it is dinner time and if it lands in the green area it is not dinner time. 'Dinner time' necessitates the child who asked the question 'feeding' one of his cardboard children into the mouth of the stand-up cardboard Mr Wolf! Insey Winsey Spider involves realistic plastic spiders that climb up a drain pipe and can be washed down again according to whether the dial lands on rain or sunshine.

Following on from there, Jumble Sale, Tummy Ache and Racing Home (Kiddicraft) and Scaredy Cat, Huff Puff and Cat and Mouse (Orchard Toys) are all well thought out and entertaining games.

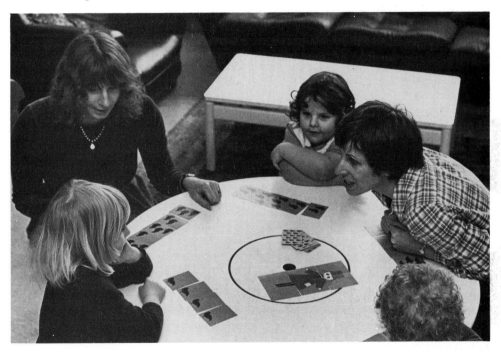

The illustration shows our language group playing Scaredy Cat. The idea is to collect as many birds as possible before the scarecrow is built. If you pick up a cat you lose all your birds — hence the name of the game.

As well as encouraging the more straightforward skills such as counting, games are a useful way of teaching a child to 'think', i.e. to hold several rules in his head, to understand the relationship between events, to note his performance in comparison with the others playing and in some cases to make choices about the most effective strategy for winning the game. In Huff Puff, for example, if he throws a wolf he can choose which of the other players' houses to blow down, with it obviously being to his advantage to blow the most advanced house down.

All these games are relatively inexpensive and can provide a lot of fun and learning. Another advantage of using them is that they are a good way to teach children to play co-operatively. This can take time with inexperienced children but once they begin to enjoy playing games and come to realise that other children are a necessary part of this enjoyment, there is often an improvement in co-operative behaviour. Mothers who use the Toy Library have often found these sort of games a useful way of getting other members of the family, especially brothers and sisters close in age, to play with the handicapped child.

Constructional Toys

More sophisticated constructional toys do require a high degree of planning, imagination and manual dexterity so for one or other of these reasons many slow developing children find them difficult, unrewarding toys to play with. When choosing constructional toys, therefore, be careful to match them as far as possible to the child's capabilities and needs. For children with good planning and imagination but poor hand and finger control, toys that fit together relatively easily such as Lego and Sticklebricks are preferable to those requiring more complicated methods of assembly. If, on the other hand, a child has quite good manual dexterity but could not follow or develop a plan for building a specific item, something like Octons (Galt) which are visually attractive, will give him practice at fitting and need only be built into abstract structures, would probably suit him best.

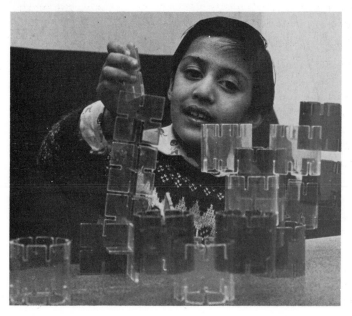

If presenting the Octons for the first time it is a good idea to build up a base yourself and then get the child to fit pieces on. This toy requires quite good handling co-ordination and involves the child in having to match up the slot on one piece with a slot on another piece and insert it at right angles. You will either have to hold the piece he is building onto steady or teach him to hold it himself. If your child is very heavy handed or destructive, more durable plain plastic octons are available but the ordinary translucent octons are more attractive. You may have to guide his hand several times before he is able to slot the pieces together for himself. At a later stage you can also play colour games with the octons, such as building a structure all in one colour or alternating two colours.

Another good toy for encouraging fine finger and hand control without necessarily involving complex planning is Constructo-Straw. It is quite difficult to fit together and will probably require some help from you at first. Different lengths of straw are included in the set. The shorter straws are easier to start with because the child can have more control as he tries to fit the straw on to the pronged wheel. With the longer straws show him how to hold them near to the end that he is going to be fitting.

A very simple construction toy that is also a fascination and cause-and-effect toy is the marble run. Several similar plastic versions of this exist (e.g. Kiddicraft 'Builda Helta Skelta'). The identical plastic pieces plus bases and supports can easily be stacked on top of each other or in more complicated patterns to form a zig-zag pathway that the marbles run down. This toy is ideal for children who are poor at constructional type play. Start with two bases and demonstrate to the child how to put the first few pieces on. Then hand him a piece in the correct orientation and either guide his hand to put it on or point to where you want him to put it. If he loses interest, show him how the marble will run down and, hopefully, this will be an incentive for putting more pieces on. When he can stack pieces easily, get him to look for the hole at one end of the piece and teach him that each time he puts a piece on, the hole has to be at the opposite end to the piece before. (This may be too difficult a skill to teach some children at this stage.)

Once built, the marble run also serves as an excellent language toy. It is good for introducing the word 'go' and for teaching the child to say something approximately like 'marble' when he wants one. If you grab the marbles as they come to the bottom of the run you then have control of the supply for games like this. You can also use forced choice questions:

'Would you like a blue or a green marble?'
'Would you like two or three marbles?'

It is also a useful toy for teaching turn taking and co-operative play. A game many children enjoy playing is for one person to put a finger in front of the hole on the top run whilst the other piles as many marbles behind the finger as possible and then shouts 'go'. At this point the other person removes his finger and the marbles all rush off down the runway.

Picture Matching

There are many games involving picture matching, many being in the form of Picture Lotto or Picture Dominoes. Giant Picture Lotto by ESA has clear brightly printed pictures in sets of four on strong wipeable cardboard; other useful lottos to follow on from this are the Galt Picture Lotto and Find It, and the Four to Eight graded series of lottos and the Dick Bruna Lotto. When it comes to dominoes the ESA Giant Picture Dominoes and the Galt Picture Dominoes and probably the best to start with.

Other useful toys for picture matching are the ESA Giant Snap Cards and the Four to Eight Identification Box. The ESA Giant Snap Cards are in fact identical to those on the Giant Picture Lotto and are a useful way of familiaris-ing a child with the pictures and the idea of matching pictures before going on to the lotto.

The Four to Eight Identification Box at £9.45 plus 70p for each strip of pictures involves a significant outlay and is best suited to the needs of a nursery or class where it will get extensive use. It consists of a long wooden box which has alternative five and ten slot lids depending on the complexity of the pro-gramme to be fed in. The programme is a strip of five or ten pictures which slide into the top of the box behind the slotted lid. Matching picture cards can then be posted through the slots adjacent to the relevant pictures. Cards are grouped in series such as toys, furniture, clothes, etc. The Identification Box is useful because it lays out the task clearly for the child and cuts down the amount of disruption or chaos that can be caused to the material by a fiddly child. The novelty of posting the pictures into the slots also keeps up interest and motivation for some children. The disadvantage of this is that the child's correct or incorrect response 'disappears' through the slot and is no longer there as reminder of what he has done. Where possible prompt him to put the picture into the correct slot and stop him from making a mistake.

Picture matching is always easier if a child lays the cards out on the floor or a table as he will be able to see the pictures more clearly than if he is waving them about in his hand. Try to have the pictures far enough apart to form two distinct groups but near enough together for the child to compare pictures easily (about 6-12 inches). The ESA Giant Snap Cards have been lent out from the Toy Library far more often for picture matching games than for actual Snap, and once a child has picked up the basic idea of picture matching this should make the introduction of picture lotto much easier, especially if you use the compatible ESA Giant Lotto and Snap. When matching pictures, get him to hold his card underneath each of the laid out cards in turn and when he finds the one that matches, to put his card *on top* of the other rather than next to it. He will then do this automatically at the picture lotto stage. For lotto you should hand him the cards one at a time and encourage a careful look around the board before putting it on, as some children soon pick up the idea that they have to put a card on the board but do not always realise they have to match it to a specific picture. Sometimes verbal cues such as 'no', or 'look for the cat' can be helpful. When he can match on to the four picture board successfully, give him two boards next to each other or introduce another simple lotto like the Galt one which has nine pictures per board. This requires more scanning and even children who have been picture matching fairly well can deteriorate in performance unless given sufficient prompts to scan the board adequately.

Picture dominoes seems to be a much harder game to teach many children. This may be more to do with the difficulty of getting them to understand what is involved in playing the game rather than a straightforward inability to match the pictures. The child has to learn that he must look at the pictures at either end of the line and scan his own dominoes to see if he has a matching picture. Many children become confused and will pick out a picture that matches the inner picture on the end domino. They also find it difficult to scan both ends and remember what the two pictures are whilst they look through their own pictures. Even when they select a domino with the appropriate picture they will quite often place it the wrong way round so the matching pictures are not together. So what is a seemingly simple game to an adult can be initially quite a complicated game for a child and underlines the need to appreciate all the things a child has to learn in a situation that we take for granted.

Thinking and Concepts (i.e. Cognitive Skills)

As well as being able to sequence and plan his activities a child needs to develop a good auditory and visual memory and to acquire an understanding of the relationship between things and an ability to predict the likely outcome of events (i.e. if I pull this saucepan down I may get burnt). To make all the input he receives manageable and useful he needs to learn to select the relevant cues in a situation and be able to categorise the information in a meaningful and accessible way (e.g. round vessels with handles are for drinking out of).

Informally many of these skills will be used and acquired by a child in his day-to-day activities but to ensure their transference to activities like reading and writing he may need to learn them in more formal ways as well, particularly if he is handicapped in some way and unable to pick out the salient points for himself so easily.

LDA have a whole series of cards and games designed for this purpose. Their 'Sound Lotto', for example, teaches a child to link familiar sounds to pictures as part of an enjoyable game. Another LDA game that is very popular is called 'Picture Clues'. Picture cards are hidden one at a time in a cardboard wallet that has several flaps with increasing size holes. The child opens one flap at a time exposing more of the picture on each turn until he can guess what the picture is. This helps to teach him that by looking at part of an object he can discern distinctive features that will give him clues as to what it is.

LDA card sets that have been popular in the Toy Library include:

'What's Wrong Card'	Pictures of silly things like a bird flying upside down or a bridge with water running over it. *Use* to develop a child's thinking skills. The mistake can be explained verbally or pointed to by a non-verbal child.
'Sequential Thinking'	Series of cards from two to several telling a story or event, e.g. a candle being lit. *Use* to teach the relationship between events in time, e.g. a match is struck before a candle is lit.
'Classification of Objects'	Cards of six different groups of objects such as flowers and dwelling places. *Use* to teach the concept of objects belonging to groups because of specific features they share (e.g. all have walls, doors and roof, all have stem and petals).
'Classification by Use'	Ten sets of cards with the objects in each set, although physically dissimilar, sharing a common usage or situation (e.g. roads, keys, tyre, petrol pump, all relating to motoring). *Use* to learn to think at the abstract level of how things are associated by usage than just by appearance.
'Things that go Together'	Pictures of objects that are associated in usage such as hammer and nail or key and keyhole. *Use* as above.
'Visual Recall Cards'	Cards with two to five symbols or pictures on them, with response cards for the symbols. *Use* to test and improve visual recall of sequences. Non-verbal children can make their responses by laying out the symbol response cards in the correct order.

With each set of LDA cards there is a leaflet describing in detail how the cards can be used at various levels, what skills they should encourage and advice on additional activities to back this up. Thus they are a useful source of ideas and information on further activities.

The skills encouraged by these cards can be backed up by a number of games; for example, getting the child to sort a whole range of objects first on the basis of size (big or small) then colour (red or yellow) and finally some other factor such as usage. A traditional memory game is Kim's Game where a tray of objects is presented and then covered up: see how many objects the child can recall with your help and a few clues! Similarly, objects can be laid out in a row, then covered, and the child asked to name them in the correct sequence. Another popular game is to hide a familiar object in a drawstring bag and see if he can guess what it is by feeling it.

Galt have an attractive association lotto called 'Find It'. There are four boards with scenes of the kitchen, bathroom, playroom and garden, and blank spaces down the sides of the boards for small cards. Each of the small cards has one of the objects in one of the pictures on it, although it is often a different size or in a different orientation so the child cannot make a direct picture match. The idea is for the child to think about which room he is most likely to find a saucepan or a toothbrush in. Along similar lines is 'Pair It' (also Galt). It has four boards of nine pictures and the child has to pair the logically appropriate card to the picture such as the arrow to the Indian or the tennis balls to the racquet. Another set of cards by Galt are the 'Odd Man Out Strips' where the child has to pick the one object out of the room that does not belong. These are another way of teaching a child about categories and are graded in difficulty so you can start with fairly concrete categories such as fruit and vegetables and go on to more abstract ones such as things that float on the sea as opposed to flying in the air.

Should you find that a child does not respond well to the cards, it may be because he does not really know what is required of him. Practical demonstration and example may be needed. With the classification by use cards a child can be given practical experience of sorting familiar household objects into piles by use. For example, you could try putting all sorts of eating utensils in one pile and washing utensils in another. Start with one object in each pile then present the next one asking the child, 'What do we do with this?' When he says 'eats' (or whatever), and this may need prompting, point out which of the other objects is also used for eating and get him to place them together. With a non-verbal child mime the activity and if possible get him to mime it as well. Then point to the other same use object and mime what is done with that. You will find that most of the LDA cards are graded in difficulty so you can start with easier examples and progress to more difficult ones.

Jigsaws

For many children jigsaws seem to have an optimum amount of enjoyment when they are not too hard and not too easy: an obvious statement perhaps, but one we need to bear in mind when choosing for a particular child. Once he has mastered the insets and sample jigsaws described in the *Toddlers* section, it is time to introduce slightly more difficult interlocking jigsaws. As mentioned before, the Giant Floor Jigsaws are ideal for this and can be followed by more complex floor jigsaws such as 'Jungle' and 'Woodland' by Galt (15 pieces) and 'Autumn', 'Playtime', 'Forest' and 'Harbour' by ESA (20 or 25 pieces), and 'Summer, Winter, Autumn, Spring' by E.J. Arnold. Of the smaller interlocking jigsaws, the 25 piece 'It's Fine Outdoors' jigsaws by Galt, the 25 piece 'Summer Day' jigsaws by ESA and 25 piece Transport jigsaws by Four to Eight, are all attractive and mounted on wood for relatively easy handling.

Children vary quite a lot in the strategies they adopt for doing puzzles. Some will collect all the pieces together in groups such as the sky or the sea whereas others will search for a specific piece to fit each time or will assemble all the edge pieces first. It does not really matter what strategy the child develops as long as it is reasonably effective. What is important is that he does not just try pieces completely at random and give up because of lack of success. If necessary, teach him whatever strategy you think he will find easiest to cope with and help him to think logically about what he needs to do:

'See if you can find the girl's coat'.
'What colour is her coat?'
'That's right, it's red. So you need to look for a red piece.'

Imaginative Play

Between three and five years imaginative play becomes extensive and elaborate. For convenience it can be divided roughly into two areas. There is play centred around model toys such as farms, hospitals, garages, dolls' houses; and play that involves the child in taking a role or pretending to be either a real or imaginary character. The kind of imaginative play and the frequency of it varies enormously between children and there is also a lot of graduating between the two areas of imaginative play. For example, a little girl may play with a doll and at the same time pretend to be her mother.

The range of good model toys is vast and choice is largely a matter of judgement of what will suit a child best and give him most play value. Some children tend to be 'object' orientated and like realistic models but do not show a great deal of imagination. Models with a lot of working parts such as the Fisher-Price Garage, Play Family Airport or Lift and Load Depot, or the Palitoy Rescue Centre may be more appropriate for these children. For those who are less interested in working models but have a fertile imagination, models that are more open-ended and have a less specific range of activities will probably be of greater play value. Here the traditional farm set or dolls' house comes into its own. As a basic dolls' house, Fisher-Price produce an attractive Play Family House and also a very colourful and interesting Play Family Village, both of which can have additional play family sets added to them. For a first train set there is the Playcraft train set in plastic, fairly durable and good value for money. Four to Eight have a reasonably priced 200 set (around £3.10) which includes wild animals, fences, trees and a mat with printed layout and also an extensive farm animals set. An unusual toy is a strong cardboard magic theatre that has people with magnetic bases who can be moved around the stage from underneath by sticks with magnets on them (ESA).

For role play, if you want something more elaborate than old curtains or mother's cast-off shoes, there are available all sorts of garments, helmets and outfits for dressing up, and props like tents and Wendy houses. Galt and ESA both have a wide range of articles for domestic play. Fisher-Price have recently brought out a medical kit and a tool kit both with some working gadgets and a carrying case. If you have a child with good understanding of language who still does not seem to indulge in much imaginative play, it is possible to inject some imagination into his play by a question or suggestion at the right time. If he is playing with the Rescue Centre, for example, you could ask him who he is going to rescue and help him build up a story of why he needs rescuing. You might have an actual model who could be stuck in the sea (piece of blue paper) or on a mountain top (upturned cup). Again, with a model farm if he is merely lining up the animals, suggest that it is feeding time and give him the model woman with the bucket to feed them. To encourage role play assign him a role such as 'Daddy' and suggest he does something that he has seen Daddy do like driving the car or digging the garden (washing up?).

Some children get so hooked on the mechanics of playing with working models that it is hard to intervene and suggest something more creative, and it may be more productive to introduce imaginative play mainly through role play and fairly inanimate material like a set of model people and wooden houses.

This may seem a rather short section for such an important area of play but once a child has started to play imaginatively, as long as he has the props and is given the occasional suggestion, he should make good progress, and too much adult intervention may not be welcome. Obviously the more events he watches and is included in, and the more outings and experiences he has, the more material he will have for his imaginative play, and he can be reminded of things he has seen and heard.

Social Play

Whereas social play as a toddler was largely confined to accommodating adults, the pre-school child now begins to learn to mix with other children and to abide by general rules such as waiting his turn. All children vary a lot in how sociable they are and handicapped children can range from the very sociable, almost 'overfriendly' child to the very withdrawn child who deliberately avoids interaction with others. Some children show good social play with their family or with their caretaker or teacher, but almost no social play with other children.

A first step is to get him playing socially with you or other closely involved adults. Some children are very specific in who they will play with and if this is the case, try to encourage him to play with other familiar adults. Brothers and sisters, depending on age and their relationship with the handicapped child, may be a good introduction to playing with other children, but not necessarily so. A playgroup or nursery is the usual way of encouraging social interaction at this age. Some children take a long time to mix but get a lot of enjoyment and stimulation from watching the other children. In some instances, where a child clearly shows interest in the others, it is not so much shyness as a lack of the necessary skills that holds him back from joining in. Some home preparation, e.g. of sand and water play, may help the socialising process; or practising with similar toys to those used in the nursery. Likewise with activities, it is possible to rehearse rhymes or actions they do at the group or movements to music. This way he will have a repertoire of behaviour that will at least allow him to play alongside the other children. At the sand or water tray, for example, this sort of situation usually leads to some social interaction even if it is only at the level of finding out that you sometimes have to wait for the implement you want or that other children do not take kindly to having things snatched away from them. Understandably, because some handicapped children are slower to learn about things like turn-taking, you may find a child throws tantrums or is aggressive with others. Most nurseries and playgroups are good at coping with this and it is surprising how often even a very difficult child settles in and learns to take his turn at things like the slide or see-saw and follow general routines such as sitting down at milk time.

Once a child is playing reasonably well alongside other children you can try and encourage more positive interaction. Either the nursery staff or the parents (or both) can provide individual preparation for group games; the important thing is to make sure that he has the necessary skills to join in, by giving him extra help and practice before putting him in the group situation.

Language Play

It is apparent by now that a child will be getting a lot of language practice through many aspects of play, particularly the areas like games, social and imaginative play. As stressed in the *Toddlers* sections, the important thing is to make sure that the child is increasing his understanding of language rather than just being urged to say words. Many of the activities and toys already suggested in this chapter will help both understanding of language and speech. In the normal child there is a lag of a few months between his understanding a word and his using a word and in some handicapped children this lag may be longer.

By this stage the child should be able to relate two named objects, like 'Put the spoon in the cup'. This ability usually occurs at around the same time as the ability to match a small toy to a picture (e.g. model car to picture of car). With increasing memory he should be able to carry out instructions which involve going to another room to fetch one or two items. Later he should be able to select objects by more indirect means than a verbal label. He might, for example, be asked to select an object by use, e.g. which one do we eat with?

Some handicapped children seem to learn to use nouns (labelling words like Daddy, Mummy, car, teddy, etc.) but take a long time to move on to using verbs (action words like walk, talk, etc.). LDA have a series of 'Action Cards'. Set 1 has four different people doing a variety of activities such as running, walking, swimming, and so on. In Set 3 each picture also includes an object so a person is doing something like watching television or brushing her hair. Set 2, which is in fact the most complicated set, includes people doing something to an object but also with a background, e.g. a woman taking a jar out of a cupboard, two children feeding two ducks on a pond. They also have a set of photographic action cards similar to Set 1.

For a non-speaking child, show him the pictures and comment on the *action* rather than labelling the person (e.g. she's swimming, she's eating, etc.). Get him to do the action as well if possible. Lay the cards out according to action and encourage the child to put further cards of the same action next to each other so he ends up with all the people swimming, eating, etc. in their own groups. For a verbal child, when you show the picture, ask something like 'What's she doing?' Children at first tend to label and say 'girl', 'man', etc. Reply, 'Yes, it's a little girl. What's she doing?' If he still does not reply appropriately, answer yourself, 'Yes, she's swimming'. When he can say what most of the people are doing you can with some cards also introduce an object, e.g. 'He's washing his hands', 'He's eating a sausage'. You may have to do this in two stages. Ask as usual what the person is doing. When he replies, 'Eating', ask 'What's the man eating?' If he says 'Sausage', you can then say, 'Yes, he's eating a sausage. What's he doing?' and, hopefully, you might get 'Eating a sausage' back. Do not correct poor articulation and accept any reasonable attempt that can be understood.

The next set of cards (Set 3) which all include a subject and an object can be used to carry this on.

Further Language Materials

LDA also have sets of cards for encouraging prepositions (on, in, behind, under) and opposite concepts (big/small, fat/thin). Again these can be used both for receptive and expressive language (understanding and speaking language).

The Galt 'Say What You See', which consists of pairs of pictures with deliberate differences graded in terms of linguistic difficulty, is a useful game. Unless very fluent, however, children tend to flounder without additional help. Non-verbal children can point to the differences but the difficulty for most children is the need to structure a long and complicated sentence to explain them. Start with the easiest picture and ask him to point out a difference. (You can point some out for him if he does not seem to understand the idea of the game.) When he has pointed to it, if he cannot explain it in words, use some prompting to help him. For example, the cupboards are open in the first picture and closed in the second, so you might say, pointing to the first picture, 'Yes, the cupboard's open' or, alternatively, 'Is the cupboard open or closed?' When he has replied you would then go on to ask the same question of the second picture. If he got both answers right you could summarise for him, saying, 'You're right, in this picture the cupboard is . . . and in this one it's . . .?' (pause for child to fill in word). With a more verbal child you might get him to say the phrase 'The cupboard is open' or 'The cupboard is closed'. Later pictures introduce more difficult sentence structures but you can use the same form of questioning to help the child, e.g. 'Is the squirrel going *up* or *down* the tree?', 'Are the rabbits *in front* of the path or *behind* the path?'

Rather more expensive than the Galt cards but useful for a school, nursery or playgroup or to borrow to use at home is Chameleon Street by Philip and Tacey. This is a whole series of figures, houses, vehicles, and so on which can be stuck to a self-adhesive album or additional display board to make up interesting street scenes. Chameleon Street, as its name implies, is a most versatile outfit because it can be used at so many levels of language development. To start with it can be used for the child to pick out labelled pieces (e.g. 'Show me Mummy') or to name pieces himself. Progressing from this it can be used to develop many parts of speech (e.g. 'Do you want a red or a brown house?' 'Are you going to put the man in front or behind the car?' 'How many trees do you want?' 'What is the lady doing?' and so on).

Books

For a child who is not yet at the reading stage but is past the one word labelling stage, story books with activities and simple picture story sequences are ideal, especially if they relate closely to the child's everyday environment. LDA have a series of 'Help Yourself Books' about activities like dressing and laying the table. These have suggestions accompanying them graded in difficulty for children at various levels of ability. Kiddicraft have a series of attractive 'Create a Story' books which include topics like 'in the home' and 'in the country'. Several flip over strips means that innumerable pictures and stories can be made up.

Books with a story told in pictures with a small number of printed words include many of the Dick Bruna books (Methuen) and 'Picture Tales' by MacDonald. The 'Thomas and Emma' books by Gunilla Wolds (Brockhampton) are also popular, with Thomas and Emma engaged in many familiar activities such as having a bath or baking a cake. However, the local public library is the best place to discover what will interest your child, and picture books can be borrowed suitable for babies upwards.

Drawing and Creative Skills

Some handicapped children reach the stage of scribbling but are slow to progress to more constructive drawing. This may be because they have poor pencil control or because they do not really know how to set about drawing a representation of a specific thing. Activities and toys such as the Magnetic Figures and Picture Printing (Galt), Jigbits (Kiddicraft), Templates (Galt and Orchard Toys) and Playdesk (Fisher-Price) are all useful for developing drawing and creative skills.

You can encourage the child to draw by playing games where you do a circular scribble or zig-zag scribble and then hand the pen to the child to do the same. Prompt him if necessary until he can do this. Then try getting him to copy dotting the paper or doing one or two straight strokes on the paper. Draw a circle for him and tell him to give the man some eyes, and if he can do this go on to ask for a nose, mouth, ears and hair, pointing to the appropriate areas if necessary — but do not be too exacting as to position!

For children with poor pencil control a useful way to give them experience of building up a man is with the Galt Magnetic Figures. These are flat wooden shapes including faces and various square and oblong pieces that can be used for bodies and limbs. Demonstrate first, naming each piece as you put it on the board.

'Here's his head.'
'And here's his body.'
'Now what do we need now?'
'I think we need some arms. Shall we put his arms on?'
'And here's his legs, one, two!'

When you have done this remove the pieces or if there are enough sort him out a similar set and ask him if he would like to make a man. See if he can pick out the head when you suggest it and point to it or pick it out if he cannot manage. Do the same for the body and if he needs help, point to where the piece should go, or for a child that can follow instructions, give him verbal guidance. Other figures can be made up in the same way. In the illustrations a child with good understanding of language is being 'talked through' copying a model, with the occasional point to help her.

Another toy from Galt that is useful for teaching a child how to construct a picture is Picture Printing. This is an ideal first printing set as it contains just six basic shapes and four colours of ink. It has been a favourite in the Toy Library and has stood up well to wear and tear unlike many printing sets that tend to be too complicated for young children and soon get broken. As with the previous activities you should demonstrate to the child and give him help when he needs it.

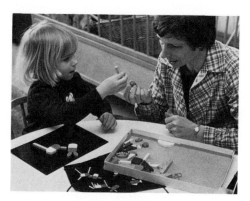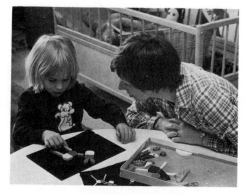

Galt have four sets of plywood templates for drawing round and Orchard Toys have three brightly coloured sets in strong cardboard. All these are suitable as an introduction to drawing round figures. Some shapes are easier than others so pick the simplest shapes initially like the Orchard Toy 'Owl' or 'Fish', or the Galt house. Demonstrate drawing round and show the child the resultant picture. It is a difficult skill for many children to acquire and you may need to guide the pencil round for him and hold the stencil still. Give as much help and encouragement as the child needs as this is a good way of building up interest and confidence in children who have experienced little success with drawing.

The Kiddicraft Jigbits consist of colourful cardboard pieces that slot together to make a variety of figures such as animals and circus characters. They could be regarded as a constructional toy but are a useful way of making a child aware of the components he needs to build up a particular model. For a start he has to sort out the pieces he needs from the whole set ('Let's find all the grey pieces to make an elephant', 'Let's find all the stripey pieces to make a tiger', etc.). He then has to learn how all the pieces are related. Children with poor co-ordination will need help in fitting the pieces together as this requires a fair degree of skill.

CHAPTER 7

Children with Special Needs

Some handicaps mean that rather than following normal development more slowly the child has to learn some skills in another way, and may learn a slightly different range of skills. A blind child, for example, will learn to make sense of his world mostly through hearing and touch whereas a deaf child will learn a lot through sight. A bright cerebral palsied (spastic) child may not be able to write with a pencil but may learn instead to type with a Possum typewriter.

Although a few specialised toys designed for specific handicaps will be mentioned in the chapter, many of the toys will be those that have already been discussed. The reason for this is that, as with most handicapped children, how you present the toy and help the child to use it is as important as the toy itself. There are some very helpful specialised toys but they are not the main resource: the handicapped child, like all others, will learn most through normal play experience with people.

Physically Handicapped Children

This is a very wide ranging group of children, from those with severe quadraplegic cerebral palsy (i.e. all four limbs affected) to those with a mild monoplegia affecting one arm or leg slightly. It is also the case that whereas some of these children will be severely delayed in development, others will be of average or above average intelligence.

This group includes children with cerebral palsy, spina bifida, muscular dystrophy and various congenital malformations of the limbs. An additional problem for some cerebral palsied and spina bifida children is that they have difficulties with the perception and integration of information. Some children, especially those with cerebral palsy, are late developing good head control and also have difficulty controlling their eye and mouth movements. Bowley and Gardner (1972) quote figures indicating that about 50 per cent of cerebral palsied children are of normal or high intelligence and the rest are below average intelligence. They also give figures indicating that 75 per cent of spina bifida children are of average intelligence with 25 per cent below average.

With a severely physically handicapped baby play that encourages head control and visual tracking and fixation is of paramount importance. Good positioning is essential. A physiotherapist or doctor can advise on this and parents may be entitled to a special form of seating or support for the child. Foam rubber play wedges or bolsters are often used as support for children with poor head control. If other sources fail, the Rubber Division of Dunlopillo will cut a foam rubber wedge to the required measurements (check with the physiotherapist what the best size will be).

With slightly older children adequate seating is also important. Specialised chairs adjustable and made-to-measure are available. These give a child support where he needs it and are designed to encourage good posture. They also have a table tray at the front which the child can play or eat on, with ledges all round to prevent objects being knocked off (*Bormobler* children's chairs, available from the Spastics Society – see illustration). Other useful chairs include the adjustable made-to-measure corner seat chair with tray fitment (J. and C. Office Furniture) and the canvas portable seat which folds flat (Temple Engineering Co.). Details of other chairs and equipment are given in *Handling the Young Cerebral Palsied Child at Home* (Finnie, 1974). Unless given advice to the contrary by a physiotherapist, a child should not be left in a special chair for long periods as he will get stiff and sore.

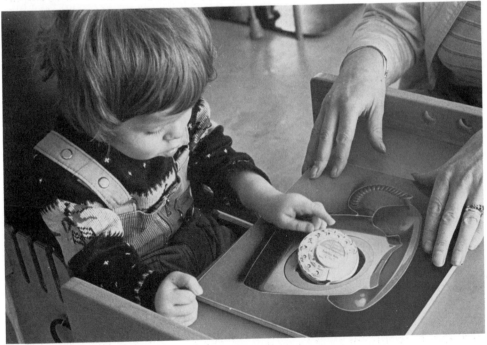

Because many physically handicapped children cannot explore their environment it is important that they be given as much experience as possible. One mother of a spastic boy used to carry him all around the house with her telling and showing him what she was doing. At the least, you should try to prop the child in a position where he can watch what is going on and he should be talked to about everyday activities such as making a cup of tea or washing up. Where possible he can be included in the experience — his hand dabbled in the washing up water or given a soft duster to grasp, for example.

The physical limitations placed on a child by his handicap differ greatly so it will be necessary to choose those activities and toys from the ones mentioned that are relevant to a child's particular difficulties. You may also need to take some of the activities and teaching techniques and adapt them to a child's specific needs. Remember that two children with the same diagnostic label can sometimes vary enormously in function depending on how seriously affected they are. The important thing is to observe what a child can do and give him help and encouragement to build on what skills he has.

For babies, the same sort of toys and techniques as those described in Chapter 3 are suitable. It is even more important that a physically handicapped baby is put in the best position for following objects and fixating objects with his eyes. Any toy that attracts a child's attention can be used to encourage head control and, by moving it, can also be used to improve visual tracking. Mobiles such as the Sleepy Time Sheep by Kiddicraft are useful as long as it is possible to put the child in a position where he can see them easily. When carrying a child around the house the mother can follow his gaze and take him up to look more closely at anything that catches his eye. Learning to hold his head up and follow people or objects takes a tremendous amount of effort for a physically handicapped child, especially those in the cerebral palsy group, so he should be given as much incentive as possible to do this. Looking up to see his mother or other members of the family is often the most powerful reward so games that capitalise on this like peek-a-boo are a priority. Following on from this games can be played involving eye-catching toys like the Playskool Flutterball or the Kouvalias toys. Move them gently in front of the child to attract his attention and then move them at varying speeds and directions to hold his interest and encourage eye following and head turning. With children who tend to look predominantly to one side (common in some cerebral palsied children), it is desirable to encourage them to turn and look in the other direction. Sitting supported by an adult or lying on the floor on his stomach are both good positions from which to encourage these activities. Some of the push- and pull-along toys on a stick such as the Wobbly Roller (Kiddicraft), Whirly Gig (Susan Wynter) and Rattle Ball (Fisher-Price) are visually very attractive, as are the pull-along Clatter Pillar (Kiddicraft) and Bob-along Bear (Fisher-Price). For a child who has such poor head control that he can only see lying on his back, it is possible to fit a sheet of perspex across the top of the cot and to roll interesting objects across the perspex.

Some children have very poor hand and arm control which severely limits their play with objects and toys. What would normally be seen as easy activities (e.g. shaking a rattle, swiping at a cradle play) requires a great deal of effort and energy. Again, it is essential to give them as much incentive as possible and to praise and encourage any attempts they make. Severely handicapped children can easily get frustrated by their fruitless efforts and will give up and be reluctant to perform physical activities. Initially toys and games should be chosen that will give a child a lot of success for a relatively small amount of effort. If the child has difficulty grasping objects start by just encouraging him to do an arm and hand swipe at objects and toys.

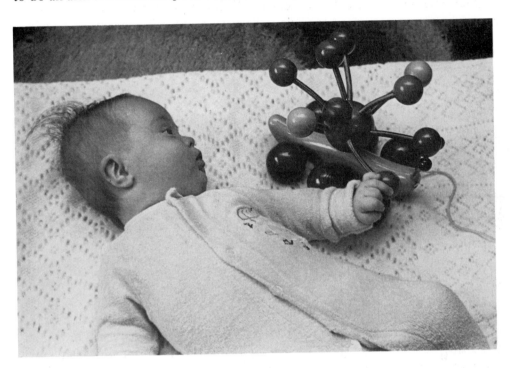

The Kouvalias toys are ideal for this as a swipe of the arm will set the balls on springs in motion. By watching the direction in which a child flails or moves his arm, you can place the toy in the path of his movement so success is guaranteed. When he can do this easily, the position of the toy can gradually be moved so he is swiping in a slightly different direction and is therefore learning to control his arm movement to some extent. Other toys that this can be tried with are the various suction rattles with wobbly tops, piled up plastic beakers or piled up material blocks. It is best not to choose things that are very solid to swipe at as the child's uncontrolled movement means that he might hit his hand hard on the object and hurt it. In the illustration Raymond has just succeeded in knocking down a stack of light foam bricks.

Even with success boredom can be a problem as, to bring about improvement in his performance, a child may have to repeat the activity many times. So the games should be varied as much as possible: for example, using the King of the Castle stacking beakers and jumping the king to the top ready to

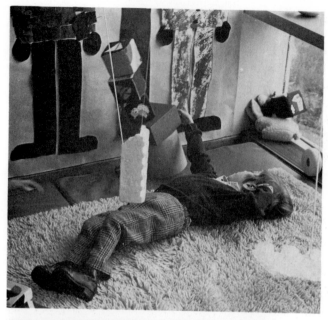

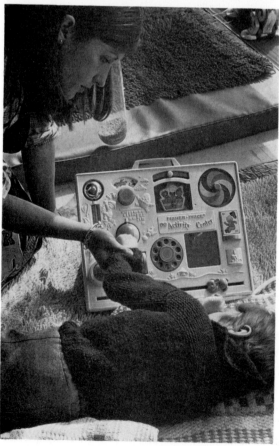

be knocked down. To ring the changes other objects such as an easter chick or a clockwork mouse can be put on top ready to be toppled. As the child's arm movement improves he may be able to direct it enough to set an object such as the Turn and Learn Activity Centre (Fisher-Price) or Cradle Play (Kiddicraft) in motion. He can be encouraged to swipe or push objects like the Flutterball, Come Back Roller or a light beach ball towards someone, preferably with an open hand as opposed to a fisted one. If necessary, his hand can be opened and rubbed or patted gently with your own open hand or on a pleasant textured surface. When he can push objects with an open hand, he can be encouraged to spin or turn objects with an open hand. The revolving rod on the top of the Playskool Activity Box is ideal for this as are the Pram People (Kiddicraft) strung on strong elastic, and later the smaller revolving drum on the Fisher-Price Activity Centre (see illustration).

Particularly with cerebral palsied children, many mothers find that the child's degree of stiffness or jerkiness varies from day to day and may also vary at different times in the same day. Many find them at their most flexible and co-ordinated when they have just had physiotherapy or have just been in the bath, so it is possible to pick a time of day when the child is at his best physically for introducing energetic play activities.

A child needs to be encouraged to feel and use both his hands as much as possible and to bring them into the midline (in front of him). He should be helped to run his hands over various textures and feel sand, water, rice, macaroni, dried peas, tissues, and so on. Some of these substances can also be sewn into small material 'feely bags'.

Another enjoyable way to promote arm and hand movements is through social play — for example, games where you both clap or raise your arms in the air or bang on the table. To increase the accuracy of these movements, the child can be encouraged to bang in a specific area or on an object like a tambourine or an upturned tin. Even when the child has his hand open, rather than clenched, reaching and grasping is a difficult skill for him to acquire, often because his inaccurate and jerky arm movements make it hard for him to get his hand in the correct position to grasp. A start can be made by handing him any of the small light rattles that he finds interesting (see p. 32) or another attractive object that is easy to grasp. With some children, at first, it may be necessary to unclench their hand in order to do this. When the child can grasp an object if it is put into his hand, the next stage is to see if he can grasp it if it is held a few inches away from his hand and later at a further distance or on the table. A two-handed grasp of objects should also be developed. Many cerebral palsied children have one hand that functions better than the other hand and, whilst encouraging him to learn further skills with his 'good' hand, he should also be encouraged to use his poor hand for more limited activities.

Another problem for many children is that their inaccurate reaching means that the toy or object they are trying to get is often knocked over or pushed out of reach. To counteract this toys should be held at the base for a child whilst he is reaching for them or toys selected that are relatively stable. It is useful to place toys which are on a slippery surface like a table on some kind of non-slip material such as the 'Dycem' non-slip plastic mat (see illustration). These are also useful for feeding because they prevent plates slipping.

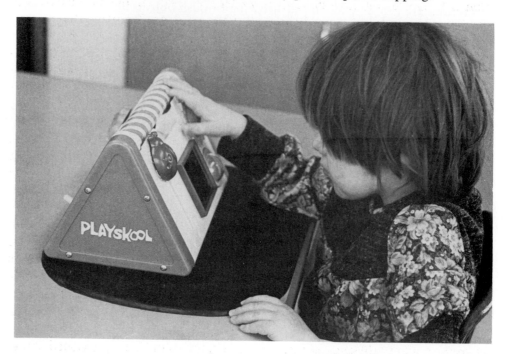

Toys that stay in place and have easily graspable handles like the Fisher-Price Pull-a-Tune Bluebird and Jumping Jack or the Kiddicraft Musical Rabbit are useful, although many children will need help with them to start with. The physically handicapped child is more likely accidentally to knock the handle and set it swinging when he tries to grasp it, so it will have to be held still for him to start with. Guidance in pulling on the handle may also be required. In the case of a toy that does not have a suitable type of handle on it, a large plastic handle called 'Simpla Pull' can be obtained from Newton Aids.

Even when a child has learnt to grasp an object fairly successfully, for some, especially in the cerebral palsied group, there is the additional difficulty of learning to release it. In all children the ability to release at will develops later than the ability to grasp, but in some handicapped children it takes much longer than usual. When a child needs extra practice in learning to release objects, you can play games where he lets go of a toy for someone else to catch or for it to fall into a bowl of water or into a large empty biscuit tin (both producing satisfying noises). To encourage early reaching and grasping it is better to provide toys and objects that can be grasped from virtually any angle, such as a crumpled tissue or duster.

Communication

Another difficulty with young severely physically handicapped children, especially where upper limb function and voice production are affected, is that it is hard to tell how much they understand because there is no easy way for them to communicate and show what they can do. Mothers often pick up clues from playing with their child and noting if he has a sense of humour or shows expectation of certain events, or eye points in an endeavour to communicate. For children where there is a marked discrepancy between their level of intellectual functioning and their level of physical functioning, this early period where no viable means of communication has been established can be a difficult and frustrating time for them. It is therefore important to make communication a priority in play and general interaction with the child. Teaching him to shake and nod his head for *no* and *yes* will make it easier to assess how much he understands, and will enable him to have some say in what he wants to do.

For the child with very poor hand and arm function, eye pointing can be of great value. Again this is useful for assessing how much the child understands. Games of 'show me the door', 'show me the window', etc. can be played, and later 'show me something red', 'show me something yellow'. You start by having a few familiar objects that the child probably knows, asking him, for example, to look at or show you the shoe. He should be praised if he looks at the right object or his attention drawn to it if he does not. You can also play games of 'where's Daddy?', 'where's the cat?', and so on. Some children find it difficult to scan so the objects should be positioned where he can see them; he can then be trained gradually to scan along a row, and later round as much of the room as possible. He can also be given practice in communicating by eye pointing — say, by your holding up milk in one hand and orange in the other and asking whether he wants 'milk or orange?'.

When a child can eye point appropriately at people and objects he can be tried out with pictures. The ESA Giant Snap cards are ideal for this. If two or three familiar pictures are laid out he can be asked to look at one of them (e.g. where's teddy?). He can also picture match if he is shown one picture and asked to select the matching one out of a row. It is necessary to have the cards far enough apart to tell which one he is looking at but not so far apart that he is unlikely to see the end card. Countless games can be played with eye pointing and brighter children can be taught to play picture lotto and dominoes using this skill. The child should be allowed to show what he wants to do by eye pointing and his interest should be followed as often as possible, as this is his only way of indicating his needs and desires.

Activities for Encouraging Further Hand and Arm Control

Moving on now to toys for encouraging hand and arm control at a later stage, the Morgenstern Arched Abacus (ESA, see illustration) is a useful toy for teaching a child to grasp and move something in a specific direction. It consists of a strong wire hoop on a wooden base with several brightly coloured balls on the wire. For a child with very poor co-ordination, you can either hold the base or use a clamp to fix it to the table. Start by having the balls at the top of the hoop and show the child how to knock them down. When he can do this try and get him to move the balls from one side of the hoop to the other. He can do this with one hand but, where possible, get him to use both hands passing the balls from one hand to the other at the top of the hoop. Children find this a surprisingly enjoyable toy, probably because the balls cannot roll away and some degree of success is nearly always possible, coupled with the fact that the balls make a satisfying thud as they land and are interesting to watch being moved around the hoop.

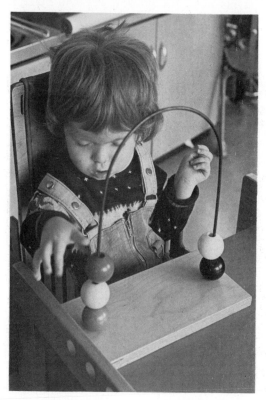

The Galt Pop-up Toy is good for encouraging both grasping and fitting. Start by holding the base firmly for the child and encouraging him to grasp the rods and take them out. Some physically handicapped children find their own solution to problems which can be very different from what you might anticipate. One intelligent but very severely physically handicapped spastic girl that I watched recently got these pop-up men out by bashing them hard with her clenched fist so they sprang out. Many children can eventually learn to put the pop-up men back in but need help and guidance to do so. If necessary, place the rod in the child's hand for him and if he cannot grasp it with his thumb and finger let him grasp it with his clenched fist with about half the rod protruding from below. Guide him physically to place the rod in the hole until he can do it for himself. If he finds this fitting task too hard try him with the ESA tunnel pegs starting with posting the rods down the funnel; details of teaching techniques for this and the Galt Pop-up Toy were given in Chapter 4 (p. 45).

The Escor toys, particularly the more stable ones like the Escor boat and charabanc, are useful for grasping and fitting, and imaginative games and sequences can be made up to hold the child's interest.

Musical toys like bells, drums, tambourines, xylophones, which involve shaking and banging are useful for developing directed movements and yet at the same time are not seen as 'hard work' by most children. Musical push-alongs like the Fisher-Price Melody Push Chime are also easy to use. Of the mechanical playing type toys the Big Mouth Singers is particularly easy to get satisfaction from, with random hitting of the keys producing plenty of sound!

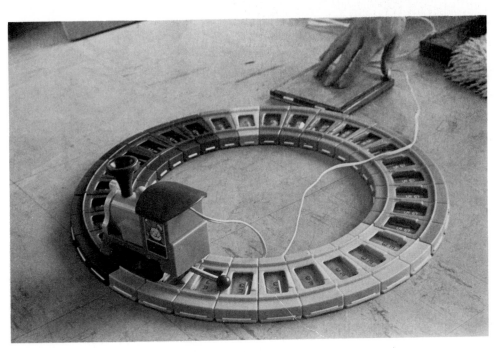

For children with very limited hand control a range of mechanised toys have been fitted with special switches. These switches consist of two large flat squares of wood joined by a hinge which when pressed together make a contact which switches the toy on. As soon as pressure is released, the contact is broken and the toy stops. The child merely needs to rest his hand or arm or foot on the wood in order to work the switch. The illustrations show the Melody train operated by a special switch, and Raymond being shown how to use a special switch to make the satellite move and flash.

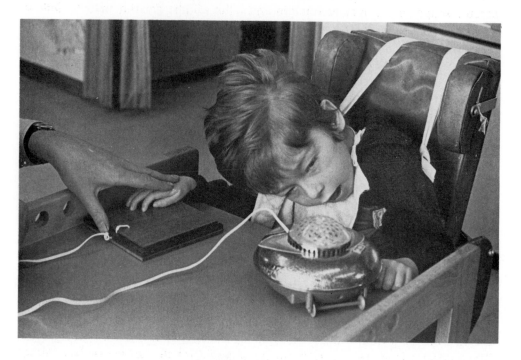

As a child's co-ordination improves either present him with slightly harder toys and activities that are still relatively easy to use for the amount of enjoyment they give, or use more complicated toys that will capture his imagination and interest, although you may in fact have to do some of the actions yourself, and help him with those that are possible for him to operate.

A toy like Farmer Giles (with animals that pop out when the keys are pressed) by Palitoy would be a good example of a toy that gives a relatively large reward for the amount of activity involved. It also allows the child gradually to improve on his own performance, so that whereas he may start by just randomly banging the keys with his fist, over time and with encouragement from an adult, he might learn to select the key he wants and press it with his fingers. Progressing on from this, the Palitoy Rescue Centre has a series of buttons that can be pushed to send plastic men hurtling down sideways into their appropriate rescue vehicles. New toys of this type come on to the market fairly often. Make sure when selecting one for a particular child that it has controls that can be worked by the child or at least would be possible for him with practice. The Fisher-Price Ferris Wheel, for example, would be fine for a child who can turn a small handle but would be very hard for a child with poor finger control and poor wrist movement.

For an intelligent child of three years or more with very poor hand function, the Kiddicraft Magic Music Maker might be useful. This is a round flattish toy with eight large keys ranged round the perimeter. Each key varies in colour and shape and is clearly numbered. A coded tune card using either colour, shape or number can be placed in the middle for the child to follow. The buttons can be pressed with fist or fingers and can be held down for as long as the child wants. After he has initially explored the toy he will probably need help to follow the coded cards, with colour or shape usually being the easiest to start with. The child may not make the connection between the coded card and its relevance to the order the keys are pressed in. Start by pointing to the first symbol on the card.

Adult: 'Look it's a blue one, Penny.
Find me a blue one (points round the keys).
Here's a blue one! (if the child doesn't find it himself).
You press it, Penny.'

If a child is very slow with this procedure, the gap between the notes may be so long that a recognisable tune does not emerge. In this case if the child is willing, take his hand and play him through the tune a few times or see if he can press the keys quickly enough if you point to the correct ones in turn for him. When he has speeded up and gained enjoyment, see if you can re-introduce following the coded cards. A rewarding toy that can be pressed with the fist but is also useful for developing finger pressing is the Pop-up-cone. Other pop-up toys can be used but make sure that the button or lever is not too stiff for the child to press.

Motivation is a big factor in how well a child learns to cope with a toy. One quite severely physically handicapped child who comes to the Toy Library has learnt how to turn the relatively stiff knobs on the Fisher-Price television for herself because she enjoys watching and listening to it so much. Children vary a lot in persistence and whereas one child can be left to struggle, another will give up almost immediately and will probably be even less inclined to persevere in the future. Unless a child is known to have good persistence and likes to do things for himself rather than have help, it is usually better to help initially and then gradually withdraw your support. Helping does not mean doing the activity for the child, it means guiding him in some way so that he learns to do the activity for himself. It is obviously more effective when the child is highly interested and excited by the activity. A game such as pushing a car hard enough and fast enough across a table so it will fall off before the waiting adult can catch it is very exciting for many children. To start with there should be one adult standing behind the child guiding his hand while the other waits to catch. As the child improves, the first adult can withdraw his help.

An exciting game for encouraging releasing might be to drop marbles in the top of the marble run. If the child is too inaccurate at first and it is difficult to prompt him to release it at the correct spot, he can be given practice with a larger target such as a sloping plank of wood. As stressed in Chapter 2 on general teaching techniques, if a child is having difficulty, either prompt him or rearrange the material or activity to make the task easier for him. This is especially important with physically handicapped children who will have to struggle to perform many activities and play with many toys. As long as a child is being constructively helped to acquire new skills, this is not giving in to him or making him lazy and might well mean that with a background of confidence and success he will be more willing to try harder activities. Having said this, it is true that there are some physically handicapped children who are good at side-tracking adults into social and language-type play to avoid engaging in physical activities. This might well be because they have gained little reward from physical activities and have often experienced failure.

Because motivation plays such a large part in what a physically handicapped child will try to do it is as well to present as large a range of activities and toys as possible (over a period of time — not all at once) for sometimes the child will play with seemingly unlikely toys and objects and perform surprisingly well. One child, for example, was observed using a large magnet (ESA and Merit) to carefully pick up paper clips from the floor.

Creative activities for physically handicapped children can start with materials like play dough and pastry which can be easily manipulated. Give him pieces to roll in his hands, press together and stick things into. Pastry cutters can be used for producing a variety of interesting shapes. Clay is enjoyed very much by some children, though others find it a bore. For children who cannot hold a paint brush or crayon, finger paints are a useful start. For older children with poor hand control, magnetic shapes such as the Galt ones are a useful way of introducing picture making as is the Galt shape printing set (see p. 116). Magnetic letters and numbers are part of the Fisher-Price Playdesk but can also be obtained separately. All these magnetic pieces will stick to a variety of metal surfaces — even a fridge or washing machine — so there is plenty of scope for artistic arrangements!

Many handicapped children besides those that are exclusively physically handicapped are poor at using both hands for co-ordinated action. Parents and teachers of handicapped children have often mentioned this as a particular area of concern, and in consequence we have built up a large repertoire of toys and activities for encouraging two-handed play, some of which will be mentioned here.

With babies you can start with simple activities such as clapping or rubbing hands together and banging two objects together, or passing a small object from one hand to the other. If necessary, place the toy in the least used hand as children will often spontaneously pass toys over to their preferred hand. When you want to encourage reaching and grasping with the non-preferred hand, place toys on the side nearest that hand, if possible out of reach of the other hand. Children will often turn their bodies in this situation in order to use their preferred hand so it is best done at a table or in a special chair where this is much more difficult to do.

Besides toys, like the ClickaWheel (Kiddicraft), which are specifically designed to encourage two-handed play, many other toys incidentally involve the use of both hands. Pushing a Jack-in-the-box back, riding a bike, rolling out pastry and clicking a toy camera, all involve using two hands. Notice how in the illustration Matthew is having to use both hands in a co-ordinated activity to push the Burbank Jack-in-the-box lid down.

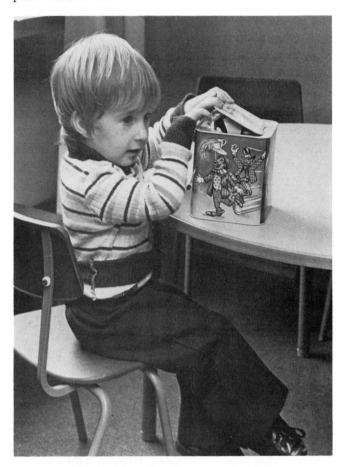

Many stacking and posting toys and puzzles need the child to hold the main part of them still whilst pieces are fitted in or on with the other hand. Likewise, many wind-up musical and mechanical toys need to be held in one hand whilst the other hand turns the knob, handle or key.

Table 7.1: Toys for Encouraging Two-handed Play in Babies

Toy	Supplier or Manufacturer	Activities Encouraged
ClickaWheel	Kiddicraft	Hold and rotate hands.
Leybourne Mirror Frame	Four to Eight	Hold in two hands.

Table 7.1: Continued

Toy	Supplier or Manufacturer	Activities Encouraged
Giant Snap Lock Beads	Fisher-Price	Pull apart, later fit together.
Rock a Stack	Fisher-Price	Hold rocking base still whilst taking off and putting on pieces.
Flip Fingers	Kiddicraft	Hold in one hand, flip twirling parts with the other.
Bird Rattle	Playskool	Hold in one hand, flip twirling parts with the other.
Tilting Tabby	Playskool	Hold in two hands.

Table 7.2: Toys for Encouraging Two-handed Play in Toddlers and Pre-school Children

Toy	Supplier or Manufacturer	Activities Encouraged
Threading beads	ESA and others	Threading.
Billie and his Barrels	Kiddicraft and various	Screw and unscrew.
Twist n' Turn	Kiddicraft	Screw and unscrew.
Flootatoota	Kiddicraft	Fit pieces together.
Nesting Eggs	Playskool	Take two pieces apart and put together.
One Dozen Eggs	Palitoy	Take two pieces apart and put together.
Screwing Rod	Galt	Screw and unscrew.
Pop-up Toy	Galt	Hold base still whilst fitting men.
Jack-in-the-box	Various, including Fisher-Price and Burbank	Activity varies according to type.
Radio	Fisher-Price	Turn stiffish knob.
Two Tune Music Box TV	Fisher-Price	Turn stiffish knob.
Pocket Camera	Fisher-Price	Hold camera steady with two hands and use one finger to click.
Triola	Galt	Hold in one hand and blow, using other to press keys.
Rolling Pin	Galt, ESA or other	Holding ends or handles of rolling pin whilst rolling out pastry.
Bicycle	Any, but check stability.	Holding on to both handle bars.

Table 7.2: Continued

Toy	Supplier or Manufacturer	Activities Encouraged
Tool Bench/Tool Kit	Playskool, Fisher-Price	Holding nuts, screws, etc. in one hand whilst using tool with other.
Escor Constructional Toys	Escor	Holding part of toy in one hand and screwing nuts with the other.
Constructo-Straw	ESA	Fine co-ordination between both hands.
Stencils	Galt, ESA, Orchard Toys	Hold with one hand, draw with the other.
Labyrinth	Brio, ESA	Careful control by twisting knobs and guiding ball through labyrinth without falling down holes.
Co-ordi	Four to Eight	Careful movement of two knobs.
Musical Slide	Matchbox	Hold base with one hand, turn handle with the other.
Mr Climb	Susan Wynter	Tug alternately on two knobs to make clown climb up string.
Tray Jigsaws and Insets	Galt, ESA, Four to Eight and others	Hold tray with one hand and fit pieces with the other.
Easy Grip Scissors	ESA	Cutting paper, etc.

For children with very limited use of one of their hands, start with toys that do not require complicated hand movement such as the Tilting Tabby which is merely held by both hands. You may have to place one of the handles in the child's poorer hand and show him how by tilting the tabby he can produce interesting effects.

Another way of utilising the poorer hand is to get him to hold the base of things still with it. For a child who can use a fist but has a poor grasp, you can start by getting him to rest his fisted hand on an inset to hold it still while he fits pieces in. You may have to physically prompt this or remind him a great deal before it will become a natural activity. Praise him whenever he does it and try to prompt unobtrusively. If he gets upset it is usually best not to persist but to find other activities that will involve using both hands. For example, large activities such as riding a bike which do not require particularly skilled use of the hands are also very successful with many children, probably because of the high motivation value and the inherent need to use two hands.

Deaf Children

Deaf children vary greatly in the degree and type of hearing loss they have, from those that are profoundly deaf to those with mild hearing loss. As soon as there is some cause for concern or a definite diagnosis of deafness has been made, a peripatetic teacher of the deaf visits the home on a regular basis. He or she will usually give information on the child's type of hearing loss, and as well as working with the child, will give advice on the best ways of helping and stimulating him. Nearly all the toys mentioned in the earlier developmental chapters will be of use but expecially those in the language and imaginative sections.

The teacher will probably advise on how to get the child's attention and the need to speak to him clearly. With profoundly deaf children it may be necessary to let them know what they are expected to do by clear points and gestures. Early social play is of vital importance because it will teach the child to look and listen. It is always necessary to make sure you have his attention before speaking to him and to keep the message as clear and simple as possible. What has to be developed first is the child's *understanding* of language rather than speech. Many of the imaginative toys mentioned before are ideal for doing this. One little deaf girl learnt what 'down' meant by playing a game with an adult where they took turns to drop a weeble down the slide, with the adult saying 'down' loudly and clearly to her and then getting her to release the weeble when she said 'down'. An added difficulty for the deaf child is that he has to look up and switch his attention away from a toy or activity in order to share it with an adult, whereas a hearing child could carry on playing whilst his mother said something like 'That's a good boy, you've got the right one'. This is another reason why social play where the child is already attending to the adult is important, particularly with deaf babies and toddlers. It is also important that they are placed in a position where they can see what is going on and hear their mother talk about what she is doing.

Many deaf children have to be taught to listen with what hearing they have. As well as doing this through normal play activities such as listening to the door bell or telephone, play can also be used. The child's attention should be drawn to sounds and he should be taken to the source of sounds so that he can see and feel the object in question. Useful toys to start with are louder rattles and music-making instruments like bells, tambourines and maracas. (See section on music-making toys, p. 42.) When he begins to show interest in the noises these toys produce, you could then, for example, see if he will imitate you in banging or shaking a toy quickly or slowly, or loudly or quietly; alternatively you could have two different sound producing toys like drill bells and a tambourine behind a screen and see if he can shake the same one as you. Moving on from this, musical toys like the Big Mouth Singers (Palitoy), Musical Radios and Ferris Wheel (Fisher-Price) and Musical Slide (Matchbox) are all attractive toys to get him to listen to. Play games where you clearly indicate to him with a visual sign when the music stops and starts.

Even with bright deaf children the lack of language can mean that they take longer to learn about concepts such as size, colour and shape. This is why it is useful to introduce these through simple clear activities (e.g. matching different colour cups to different colour saucers) that can be understood without verbal explanations, after a clear demonstration has been given. One or two new words such as 'red' or 'stir' could then be introduced in this situation. However, it is important that in our concern for producing language, we do not in fact end up doing things that are less likely to produce language. Recent research at Nottingham seems to indicate that placing emphasis on language for its own sake rather than as a part of meaningful communication (i.e. a normal two-way conversation) tends to inhibit rather than help produce language. It appears that deaf children, like most other children, are quick to realise when language is being used to 'test' them rather than as a genuine communication, for example:

Adult: What colour's this one? (holding it out in front of the child).
Child: (no answer — carries on playing with her own toy).
Adult: It's red. Say 'Red'.
Child: (no answer).

Of course, children sometimes enjoy being told the colours of things and will point their finger to each colour in turn to indicate that they want an adult to name it. In this situation the child is showing non-verbally that he *wants* the colours named so in that respect it is a genuine communication or interaction rather than information being imposed on an unwilling recipient. Similarly, genuine communication situations will often be more productive:

Adult: Would you like to wear your blue skirt or your red skirt today?

You cannot always rely on everyday situations bringing in the words and concepts you want to introduce, and even if they do the context can sometimes be too confusing or complex. Play situations can be used here if you find activities that the child is clearly interested in and wants to be involved in.

Adult: Which little man shall we put on here? (pointing to the top of the toy slide). Shall we have the RED man or the BLUE man?
Child: (points to red man).
Adult: Oh, you want the RED man. Right, let's put him on the slide.

In this situation communication will usually come naturally and, in the long run, spontaneously. It does not matter if at first the child uses gesture, as in this example. It shows that he is listening *willingly* to what you are saying and is keen to communicate back. Rather than concentrating on the language in particular, it is better to focus on the *play situation* as a whole and let the language take care of itself.

There has been controversy over whether young deaf children should be encouraged to gesture. The fear has been that if a child is allowed to gesture or sign he will not bother to speak. Recent evidence questions this assumption and in some cases shows that letting a child learn a gestural sign system may in fact encourage spoken language in due course. The argument behind the new approach is that it is vital for a child to learn first what language is about, be this at a non-verbal level, and that once the importance of being able to communicate via language is apparent to the child there will be strong personal motivation for him to learn to speak as this is quicker, and more efficient and socially acceptable, than using a sign system or gestures.

Visually Handicapped Children

As with deaf children, visually handicapped children vary in degree and type of visual impairment from the totally blind to those with a reasonable amount of partial sight. In educative terms a line is usually drawn between those who have to be taught by non-visual methods and those who can be taught by sighted methods. The former group, even if they have light/dark perception are usually described as *blind* whereas the latter group are called *partially sighted*.

The Blind Child

Blindness, perhaps more than any other handicap, is seen as something 'special' which will require different handling, rearing and teaching to that of a normal child. Parents of young blind children are often anxious to know what special things they can do to help their child and may feel rather let down and disappointed that more specific activities are not suggested. In some cases parents are so overawed by knowing that their baby is blind that they have little confidence in their own child rearing abilities and feel that only the 'experts' know what is the 'right' way to bring up a blind child. In fact the best, but perhaps the most difficult, thing for parents to do is to treat their baby foremost as a person and only incidentally as a blind baby. This does not mean being insensitive and unaware of a child's special needs but that by knowing and relating to the baby as a person they will probably be more tuned into these than if they are constantly thinking 'what should I do for him as he's blind'. Research in this area indicates that the blind children who develop best are those from normal caring homes with warm, relaxed parenting.

Guidelines to Development in Visually Handicapped Children

Some tentative guidelines to their development can be given, though individual children vary tremendously, and the notes that follow assume children of average ability, who are not suspected of having any other handicaps.

Smiling. At about six weeks (same as sighted) but fleeting and not used as a greeting, although this develops later (maybe six months before it is similar to that of a sighted infant).

Head Control. Same as for sighted children (3-6 months).

Sitting Alone. Some as for sighted children (5-8 months), some late. Many, even when able to sit unsupported, show a preference for lying down.

Standing. At normal age.

Crawling. Late – average age is over one year – and bottom shuffling is common.

Walking Free. 1½-2½ years on average. The sighted child walks independently about three months after walking with hands held. The visually handicapped child may not do so for 8-9 months.

Language. Studies of comparison of language between sighted and blind children present a rather confused picture but overall it seems that their rate of development is about the same for the first year, but that there may be some time lag in the second year when the sighted child is rapidly expanding his vocabulary by naming things, so that whereas the sighted child is talking in short sentences by two years, the blind child, on average, is not doing this till three years.

Blind babies are almost totally dependent on their mother or other caring adults for stimulation and information about the outside world. Because of this it is essential that they have a lot of handling and cuddling and social play with caring adults. In general they are no more delicate than other babies and many respond well to active and boisterous play with trusted adults (see illustration). This should be developed gradually and not begun suddenly without giving the baby warning of some sort to cue him in to what is coming. When he is too young to understand words, tone of voice will help alert him to what is likely to happen. Tell him if you are going to pick him up or put him down and tell him where you are taking him even it is only from one side of the room to the other. If you are playing an anticipation game of 'I'm coming to get you', for example, pat or scratch your hands on the carpet as you move towards him so that he can gauge your progress. Similarly, introduce toys such as rattles gently from a distance starting with those that have soft swishing sounds rather than harsh squeaks: many blind children do not like squeaky toys so introduce them with caution.

Toys, even noise or music producing ones, do not have for many young blind children the interest they have for sighted children. Although this is

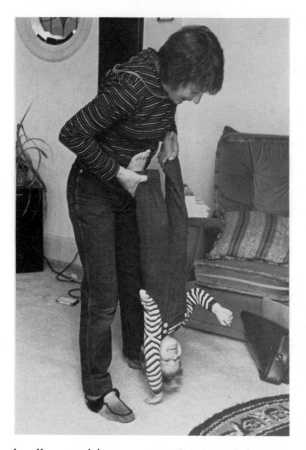

hardly surprising, as many toys must seem meaningless to the child, it is difficult in one's concern not to keep trying out and thrusting new toys on the child in the hope of engaging his interest. Many mothers have noted that their blind child would rather pick things up for himself than have them put into his hand. He may suddenly find something cold and hard or soft and furry thrust into his hand with no warning and with no idea of what arm muscle adjustments to make for the weight of the object. If he feels for objects himself he can let his hand brush against them and can then explore more thoroughly with his fingers before deciding whether to pick the object up. One mother found it useful to put her daughter in the lobster pot playpen for half an hour each day with a variety of familiar textured toys and objects that she could pick up in her own time. There was also the advantage that when she cast an object away it was not lost to her and could be rediscovered fairly easily. Like many blind children she disliked handling new toys so these were only introduced one at a time and were left for her to get used to gradually. Occasionally her mother would encourage her to pat and feel a new object. The line between leaving a blind child to experience new activities and objects and actively forcing them on him can be a difficult one to tread but most mothers seem to manage it well.

Some blind babies seem to go through a period where they play quite willingly with a whole variety of rattles and then at a later stage seem to show little interest in the handling either of rattles or other toys. This can be a disappointing time for parents as there often seems to be few noticeable signs that their child is progressing. It may well be the case that, as with sighted children, when there is often a slowing down in their language development while they are learning to walk or vice versa, the blind child is spending his time listening to sounds and language and trying to make sense of them: this occupies a lot of his thoughts and attention. If you watch a young blind child you can often see him 'stilling' to a faint background noise that a sighted child of the same age would normally ignore. Probably this pre-occupation with making sense of the auditory vibratory world plus the relative meaninglessness of many toys accounts for the lack of interest shown in toys for long periods of time by some blind children.

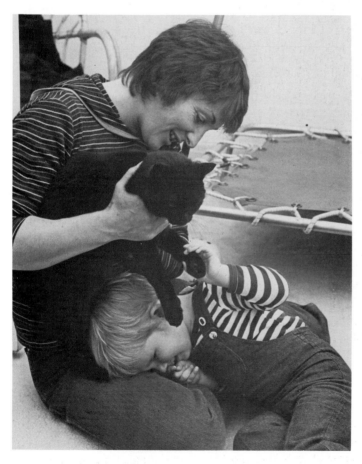

Although it is understandable that a blind child may not show interest in a lot of toys favoured by other children, this does not mean that he is not learning to explore with his hands and this should be encouraged as much as possible. Place him on different textures — rugs, furniture, grass, etc. — and also give him 'feely boards' to experience even more textures — velvet, polystyrene, sandpaper, fur, hessian, string, etc. glued onto strong pieces of cardboard. They often have quite strong preferences about the sort of materials they like to handle. Some children, for example, may only like soft materials like fur, lambswool or angora whereas others strongly dislike these soft materials and much prefer hard smooth ones like metal and plastic. Start by introducing a wide variety of the materials the child favours but gradually introduce other sorts so that he will have opportunities to learn to handle a range of different types. Sand and water play and bowls or 'feely bags' of dried peas, polystyrene chips, pearl barley, dried butter beans, etc. are also ideal for introducing new textures.

If you watch a young blind child, even if he is not handling objects and toys much, you will often notice that he frequently fingers or scratches at any surrounding textures. Take advantage of this by putting him in as many different places as possible. Sit him in the corner of the settee or arm chair and place different cushions nearby, put him on different carpets or rugs or lay him on differing bedspreads.

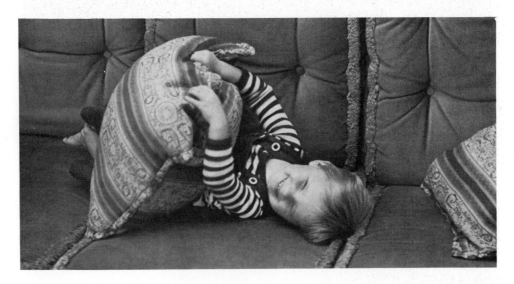

Even blind children who can sit and stand without support still seem to like lying flat on the floor at times with their face and hands in contact with the floor. The large bean and sag bags used for sitting on are often a great favourite especially if covered in an interesting material. James was recently introduced to a sag bag at the Toy Library. He showed little interest when his hand was taken to pat it, probably because this gave him little idea of the potential of the toy. His mother then placed him on it and played a game of bouncing him up and down. James was soon laughing and rolling all over it and thoroughly enjoying games of being rolled up in it by his mother. The bag has a nylon fur covering which he liked fingering and small polystyrene chips inside which made a pleasant swishing or crunching sound as James moved about on it.

It is interesting that although James is perfectly capable of sitting up that he spends a lot of time with his body in contact with various surfaces. This is common in young blind children. Notice how in the illustration he feels the radiator with his feet. His mother had observed that he often used his feet for exploration and therefore left them bare as often as possible in the house.

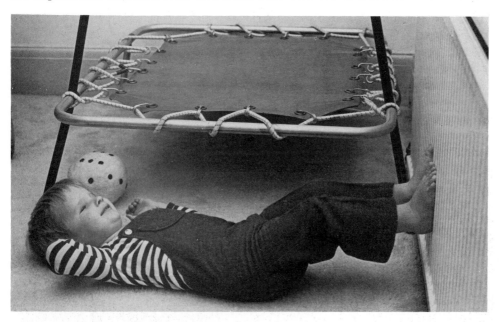

The second picture shows James exploring a small hole in a foam ball.

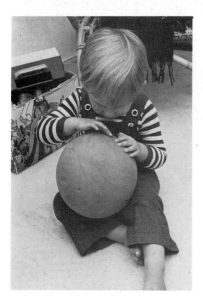

For children who are reluctant even to feel textures, the best approach is often to let them feel a variety of materials when being handled by their mother and other adults. In addition to differing clothing or putting on an apron or overall, a mother can try wearing necklaces, brooches, earrings or even a hat.

Toys for Blind Children

Having mentioned the lack of interest shown in many toys by some blind children and the overriding importance of social play, it is also true to say that some children do get a great deal of enjoyment from toys. The best ones to start with are those that make an interesting sound or have an interesting texture. A variety of rattles will give experience of many materials and types of sound production. Suction rattles that will not get lost are a good idea. Sound producing balls like the Chime Ball (Fisher-Price), Action ball (Play-skool), Musical Ball (ESA) and Discovery Ball (Four to Eight) are all suitable.

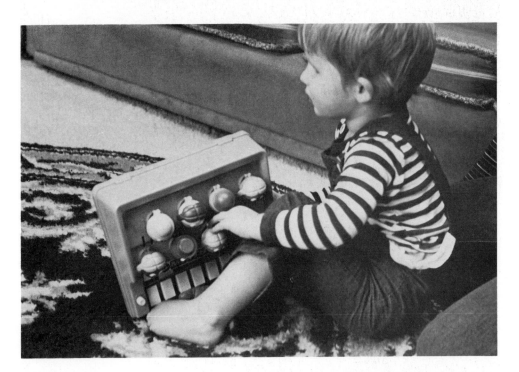

Most of the activities on the Fisher-Price Activity Centre are noise producing and this, like the suction rattles, has the added advantage of not being 'lost' if the child lets go of it. Similarly, music boxes like the Pull-a-Tune Bluebird (Fisher-Price) and Musical Rabbit (Kiddicraft) are also static, although it may be some time before a child learns to reach out and locate the handle for himself. Initially you may have to place his hand on the handle many times and show him how to pull it before he associates the pulling with music production and then learns to search for the handle himself.

At first it may be necessary to shake toys like rattles and then place them in the child's hand but later he should start to reach out when he hears the sound. This is called reaching on sound cue and usually develops in blind children between nine and twelve months, but there is a lot of individual variation and it may take another three to six months to perfect this skill. It is an important skill to encourage because it means the child can start to actively respond and reach out to stimulating events, and he is not dependent on an adult handing him his noise producing objects.

Blind children tend to be slower than sighted children in playing with toys even of the noise producing variety so that the tambourine or xylophone that is ignored at one time may be played happily with at an older age. A whole variety of music making toys are available (see Toddlers section on music making, p. 68). Wind-up and battery operated type musical toys are

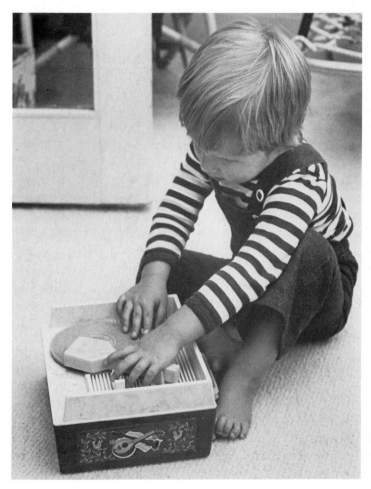

often big favourites and may be the first toys to really interest the child. James's mother found the Palitoy Big Mouth Singers (illustrated) the first toy for a long time that James had actively and positively explored and shown sustained interest in. Other musical toys that could be tried are the Fisher-Price wind-up radio and record player (illustrated), Musical Slide (Matchbox), Musical Fire Engine (Kiddicraft), Melody Train and Musical Ferris Wheel (Fisher-Price). With toys that have moving parts like the Ferris Wheel, take the child's hand and rest it on the moving parts so he can feel it going round.

A real radio or cassette recorder is often a favourite. Many blind children enjoy listening to music on the radio and the temptation can be to leave it on for hours at a time because they enjoy it so much and it seems to keep them occupied. The problem with this is that it gives the child a passive listening role and does not encourage him to be active himself. Nursery songs and games with an adult where he joins in or makes particular responses are better because they encourage him to participate and to develop meaningful language. However, it is important that he is not encouraged just to repeat phrases and jingles that are meaningless to him as this encourages a 'parroting' type of language rather than meaningful communication. Start by giving him names for things he touches: 'soft', 'hard', 'warm', and so on; and for activities he carries out: 'jumping', 'drinking'. Name objects that he regularly handles such as a cup or a spoon, rather than talking about abstract events. Constantly tell him what sounds are and take him to the source of them (e.g. to the telephone when it rings or to feel the washing machine vibrating when it is in use). Get him to feel and name the parts of his body and your body. Involve him in as many everyday activities as you can: feeling and stirring the cake mixture, holding a whole egg, listening while you crack it and then feeling the broken shells. Talk to him about what you are doing and what is going on, particularly in relation to the things he is doing – the sounds he is hearing and things he is touching. Observing a mother who was blind with her young blind child it was noticeable that she constantly spoke to him about what he was doing, even though this involved asking us first about what he was doing. 'Oh, so you've picked it up and now you're turning it round and it's got round edges and you can feel the hole in the middle . . .' and so on.

One of James's favourites toys at the moment is the Trampoline (ESA, Galt). This is an ideal toy for a young energetic blind child because it means he can let off steam and develop co-ordination and balance without the danger of bumping into things. Although blind children on average learn to stand alone at the same age as sighted children they take much longer to learn to walk free, and with many it is clearly a question of building up their confidence. Often a heavy weighted baby walker or push-along like the Mothercare lion can be useful for encouraging them to walk around the house and learn the layout, with the advantage that the walker will bang into the wall before them. Similarly a small stable trike or sit-on toy (see p. 76) is useful for exploring the house and garden.

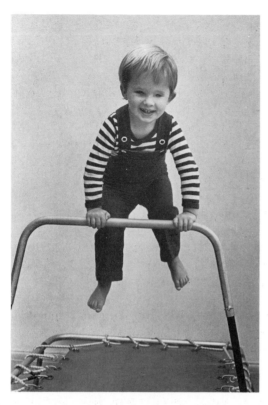

Mothers often find that their child will walk as long as he can hold lightly on to one finger or a piece of skirt. Games with two adults or with one adult and the child standing up against the sofa can be useful for building up confidence. Start by getting him to take one step into your arms accompanied by lots of praise and excitement and a jump in the air if he enjoys it. Gradually increase the distance until he is taking two or three steps using either your voice or a favourite noise producing toy as the incentive.

Models in general, like dolls' houses and farm animals, are not very successful with younger blind children because without the visual impact they bear very little resemblance to the real thing. However, larger toys like the ESA Hoover are large enough and realistic enough to be recognised as a model of a hoover and the interesting whirring sound it makes as it is pushed along also appeals to children. Another toy that has been successful with a number of blind children is the Morgenstern Arched Abacus. Because the toy is static the balls do not get lost and they make a nice clunking sound as they fall down and their movement can be followed to some extent with a hand. Likewise the Slinky makes a pleasant sound and moves in an interesting manner.

Blind children tend to be dependent on their mothers for a longer period of time than sighted children and sometimes have a number of fears such as walking on grass or going in the bath. These are usually overcome gradually and it is always best not to overwhelm a blind child by introducing too many new events or toys at once. For example, it is probably not a good idea to give him all his Christmas presents at once but to introduce them over a number of days and weeks. And the wrapping paper and string may well be a lot more fascinating than the toys themselves to start with!

Toys and Play for Pre-School and Nursery Age

With recent changes in attitude towards handicapped children, integration with normal children, particularly at nursery level, has become widespread policy in some areas. Whilst this is probably on the whole a progressive and useful move, with blind children it is somewhat questionable and each case needs to be judged on its individual merits, bearing in mind not only the facilities a nursery or playgroup can provide but also the personality of the child.

As mentioned before, many blind children are dependent on their mothers for a longer period of time and show strong separation anxiety which is quite understandable. They are also slower than sighted children in learning to play socially with other children. For many of these children a nursery, however good, can be a noisy and bewildering place that is difficult to make sense of. Some children tend to withdraw in this situation and even after a long period like a year they may be subdued and passive in a nursery type setting. So unless a child is very robust and outgoing in spirit, parents should not be pushed into sending him to nursery unless they think he will cope. If he starts and does not settle in quickly it is probably unwise to continue sending him. A blind child has so much to learn in the home environment that he may not be ready to mix with others in a large group until he is four or five. If he has no brothers and sisters other mothers can be invited round, one at a time initially, so that he can get used to playing alongside other children. If he does attend a nursery or playgroup it is better if one particular helper can be assigned to him and he can be part of a small group, with one familiar room or a corner of a large room partitioned off as a home base. To begin with his mother should stay with him until he has had a chance to get to know his surroundings and become accustomed to the noise — which may take several sessions or even longer.

More constructive activities and games involving touch can now be introduced. A number of commercial ones exist but one of the best games can be made easily and inexpensively. This is called 'feely Lotto' and works on the same basis as a picture lotto but with different textures instead of pictures. To begin with the child is simply taught to match textures with a number of individual boards with widely differing materials glued on — fur, corrugated paper, polystyrene, etc. As with picture lotto you start with just two textured cards, get the child to feel them both, and then give him a third one to match to one of them. When he can match textures individually, give him a board with four textures on it (each piece about 9 x 9cm) to match cards on to. At this stage you can try to introduce a game of lotto. Let him feel his board in front of him and let him feel that you also have a board. Then present him with a textured card and let him decide if he has a matching texture on his board. If not, let him feel that the correct texture is on your board. When he can cope with this you can go on to using a 9 card lotto or 'feely dominoes'.

ESA produce a number of toys specifically for handicapped children. Their tactile board (£10) is in fact a wooden framed version of the feely lotto described above, but can have new textures fitted. Rather less expensive are ESA's Tactile Patterns and Touch a Shape. The tactile patterns consist of eight bridges with different patterns hidden underneath and matching tablets which can be fitted to the correct bridge. This is a useful game to play with blind and sighted children together as all have to find the correct pattern by touch. The Touch a Shape boards enable the child to match pieces on by shape or texture. Another very useful toy by ESA at £3.95 is the Dunwell Frame. This has a special surface that leaves a series of raised dots when a child draws on it so he can feel what he has drawn.

Four to Eight produce two sets of dominoes suitable for blind and partially sighted children. The Shape Dominoes at £5.60 have geometrical shapes cut out of the wood. The Finger tip dominoes are rather expensive at £14.65, but are very attractive and would be useful in a nursery or toy library. Each domino has one of seven materials such as leather, felt or rubber set into it. Four to Eight also produce a touch tuner at £10.75 which again works on the same principle of matching textures as in the feely lotto, but this time they are encased in circles.

A number of toys, particularly in the inset and shape matching line, not designed specifically for blind children can be useful. Any insets with clear and well defined shapes can be used such as the Galt Traffic Tray or the Susan Wynter tea-time puzzle. A blind child is having to make a big jump to learn that three-dimensional objects that he feels are being represented in a two-dimensional manner, so these should only be introduced when he has a clear idea what the objects are and sufficient understanding of language for you to explain what the pieces represent.

For children with a good understanding of models, take apart constructional toys like the Escor 2 horse roundabout or aeroplane can be introduced. You will probably need to talk them through and help them to put them together at first but many children become surprisingly competent. Language is a big help: an intelligent blind girl was 'talked through' the assembling of a train set she had not encountered before in the Toy Library, with remarkable ease. Also useful for encouraging manual dexterity is the Playskool Take Apart Work Bench.

Imaginative play and role play is generally late in developing in blind children but is important to their development and understanding of the world. Encourage simple role play such as bathing dolly and putting her to bed. Many blind children have a good ear for imitating voices and can carry on elaborate imaginative conversations with several participants. Imaginative play is best encouraged with real objects like tins and apples and oranges for shopping rather than models.

The Partially Sighted Child

Partial sight can take a number of forms each affecting a child's vision in a different way. Some kinds of partial sight leave a child with very patchy or distorted vision so that it is difficult to envisage exactly what he sees. Often the only way to get some idea of what he can see and in what conditions is to observe him closely in a number of situations. If you lay him down does he turn his head to a light source such as a window? Does he seem to see best in very bright or rather dim light conditions? What distance is he most likely to reach and grasp a toy at? Does he follow people round the room with his eyes even if they are not speaking or vibrating the floor? At what distance can he follow a moving or dangling object with his eyes and what sort of size does the object have to be? Does he seem to see most objects within a reasonable distance or only those that are very bright or shiny? Do objects have to be placed in a specific part of the normal field of vision before he seems to notice them, that is does he only notice objects above eye level or below eye level, or to the left or the right? Does he seem to see large objects such as a chair or a person but not be able to pick out a small object like a purse or a button?

When you have a fair idea of what the child can see you can choose toys accordingly and place them in the best position for him to see. Present him with bright, clear, visually attractive objects and encourage him to use sight as much as possible. For babies, attractive rattles like the Fisher-Price flower rattle of the Playskool Happy Rattle are useful. If he can follow a moving object with his eyes the Playskool Flutterball can be tried. The Playskool Activity Centre which has a firm base and an attractive candy striped rotating rod on the top is being inspected in the illustration by Eileen who is partially sighted. Notice how she is peering closely into the mirror on the side of the centre.

The Kouvalias range of toys with their bright glossy parts are ideal for many partially sighted children. Also popular are the ESA big translucent threading beads and the bright Fisher-Price Snap Lock beads. The Fisher-Price Rock-a-stack would make a good introduction to stacking toys, while for older children the large black and white dominoes and the colour touch tuner by ESA are useful. Choose clear uncluttered pictures and insets which do not confuse a child but encourage him to make use of what vision he has.

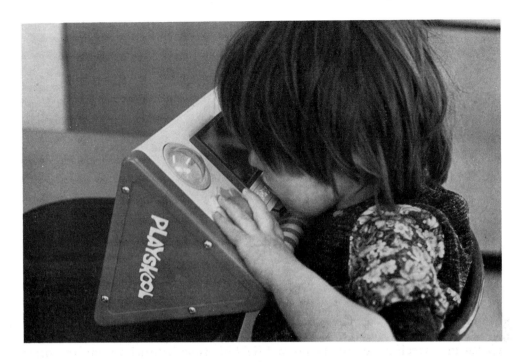

CHAPTER 8

Choosing and Buying Toys

Choosing and buying toys for special purposes is not easy. Five years of buying toys for a toy library has taught me that it takes time and effort to find 'good' toys and that it is easy to make mistakes. Nearly all the toys mentioned in this book have been used in our toy library and have stood up reasonably well to the test of time and also to the test of interest.

To start with it is worth getting hold of the main toy catalogues (list of names and addresses given in Appendix D). For younger children the Galt, ESA, Mothercare and Early Learning catalogues will give a fair range of toys. The advantage of this is that you can browse through them at home and consider carefully which toys would suit a particular child; the disadvantage being that you have not got the toy in front of you to inspect and try out. By sticking to reputable firms like the ones mentioned you can be fairly certain that the toys will be well made and designed although the larger items are sometimes rather expensive for an individual child and are better suited to the needs of a nursery, playgroup or school. The Toy Libraries Association (1981) have recently brought out a book called *The Good Toy Guide*.

An alternative to catalogue browsing is systematically to survey local toy shops. But unless there is one large and very comprehensive toy shop in your town you will probably need to go to several shops and department stores and chain stores to look at a full range of toys. For babies, larger branches of Boots and Mothercare stock a wide range, with Boots carrying a good selection of Kiddicraft Toys. Both Boots and Woolworths stock many Fisher-Price toys. Stocks of toys fluctuate according to time of year with a gradual build-up from September towards Christmas. A visit during November often gives you the best selection to choose from before the Christmas rush.

Increasingly toys are packaged in boxes which are sellotaped down. If a display toy is not available for examination ask to see one as it is impossible to judge the quality from the pictures on the boxes. One very attractively illustrated activity centre that I inspected recently literally fell apart in my hands. It was made of poor quality brittle plastic and the moving parts were not firmly joined to the main body of the toy. Before buying, try the toy out for yourself: are the controls too stiff for a child to turn? Are they awkwardly placed? Can removeable pieces be fitted back on to the toy easily?

Many toy libraries now exist. Some are for all children in an area to use and some are specifically for handicapped children (see list of addresses). New ones are opening all the time so it is worth checking with the Toy Libraries

Association to see if one is opening in your area if there is not one already. And if you know of a group of mothers who would be interested in setting up a toy library, the Association produce a pack on setting up and running a toy library and also hold training courses. Toy libraries vary considerably in the way they are run but the majority usually hold sessions on a regular basis at which parents and children can get together as well as choosing toys to borrow. Some are entirely free, others charge a small joining fee or a small amount for each toy borrowed. Even if you feel a child is 'too young' or is not interested in toys, it may still be worth checking the local toy library out because some serve as a general resource and information centre and try to give support and advice on a child's overall development. Meeting other parents can be very useful and many toy libraries have voluntary services of interested professionals like speech therapists and physiotherapists so that parents can get advice on things like seating or feeding as well as borrowing toys to take home. If a local toy library is not able to offer all these facilities, the people running it will often know who to get in touch with or where to go to obtain advice.

Parents are sometimes worried about borrowing toys from a toy library because they fear that the toys may be broken or lost, but most libraries accept (expect, if they are realistic!) that toys do occasionally get damaged or lost and would rather feel that a toy is well used than that it gets put in a cupboard and is never brought out between visits for fear of breakage. Some precautions are possible. If brothers and sisters tend to remove or fight over the borrowed toys they can be kept for a time when siblings are not around or when play can be supervised. Again, with a destructive or heavy-handed child, toys can be brought out when an adult can control their use.

When lending toys for a particular child I find it is better to provide a mixture of toys, including some he will be able to play with on his own and some that he will need help with. Not all toys conveniently fall into these categories for all children but it is a useful and practical way of viewing them. For children who are very distractable or get bored easily you can bring out one toy at a time and if the child shows interest, try and get him to play with it for a reasonable length of time in a constructive manner. It is surprising how even with a completely non-verbal child you can quickly set up the understanding that he does not get the next toy until he has done something constructive with the one he has got (e.g. finished a puzzle). This does not need to be a confrontation or bribe situation but rather a positive situation where he gets rewarded with another toy or activity for his endeavours whether these included considerable help from you or not.

Because the present range of toys is so wide some existing toys will not have been seen in our toy library. In addition to this, new toys are being produced all the time so that it is best to use this book not as a definitive work on toys but as a guide to choosing types of toys and carrying out activities. It is always useful, of course, before buying specific toys, especially expensive ones, if you can watch other children playing with them.

It is hard to make 'rules' for buying toys but here are some general hints.

(1) Choose toys by well known manufacturers.

(2) Choose toys that are flexible in having more than one use or activity.

(3) Choose different types of toys bearing in mind what the child already has so that he will be encouraged to play in a variety of ways: some toys to encourage imagination, some fitting, some cause-and-effect, and so on.

(4) Choose toys that will be of particular interest to the child (e.g. if he is interested in sound give him sound producing toys but observe him closely as it may be that he only likes certain types of sounds).

(5) Keep a list of toys you would like to get for your child and who makes them or where they can be obtained so that if relatives and friends want suggestions for Christmas and birthday presents, you have them at hand.

(6) Watch other children at nurseries or playgroups playing with toys you have not seen before and try them out for yourself.

(7) Watch out at quieter times of the year like after Christmas and during the summer months for special offers on toys. Considerable reductions are sometimes made on named toys such as certain Fisher-Price or Palitoy ranges.

(8) Club together to order toys as savings on postage or concessionary rates are often available for orders over a certain amount from catalogues.

(9) If you want advice on toys or want to track down a specific toy try your nearest toy library or contact the headquarters of the Toy Libraries Association, Seabrook House, Wyllyotts Manor, Darhes Lane, Potters Bar, Herts, EN6 2ML (Telephone: 0707 44571). The British Toy Manufacturers Association, 80 Camberwell Road, London SE5 0EG (Telephone: 01-701 7271) also run an enquiry service.

Toy List

This is not a comprehensive list of toys but covers those we have found useful in our Toy Library. Generally they are well designed, will stand up to fair wear and tear and are reasonable value for money. A few are poor in one respect, such as durability, but are included because they have considerable value in other respects. Particular assets and drawbacks of individual toys are given under the heading 'comments'.

In keeping with the preceding chapters, the Toy List is divided into the same four main areas:

Babies,
Toddlers,
Pre-school and Nursery,
Special Needs.

In the first three areas it is further divided into types of toys such as Musical or Construction, and in the fourth area — Special Needs — it is divided into types of handicap.

Toys marked with an asterisk* are those we have found *particularly* useful. Generally they have most of the following properties:

(1) Well designed.
(2) Appeal to a wide variety of children.
(3) Good value for money.
(4) Durability.
(5) Especially good at promoting one or more aspects of play.

Toys marked with two asterisks** have most of the above properties and, in addition, are those we have found *outstandingly popular* and particularly useful with children who on the whole have shown little interest in playing with toys. For addresses of catalogues, suppliers and manufacturers, see Appendix D.

Price   A: under £1   C: £3 - £6   E: over £10
Code . B: £1 - £3   D: £6 - £10

FOR BABIES

Toy	Supplier or Manufacturer	Price	Availability	Comments
Mobiles				
Cat Mobile	Mothercare	B	Mothercare Shops or Catalogue	Visual.
Musical Cat Mobile	Mothercare	C	Mothercare Shops or Catalogue	Visual and Auditory.
Nursery Mobile	Galt	C	Galt Catalogue and Shops	Bright attractive plastic shapes.
Music-Box Mobile	Fisher-Price	D	Chain Stores, Dept Stores, Toy Shops, etc.	Visual and Auditory. Animals and people move round to music.
Sleepytime Sheep (Mobile)	Kiddicraft	C	Chain Stores, Dept Stores, Toy Shops, etc.	Bright visually attractive plastic shapes.
Windchimes	Oxfam		Oxfam Shops	Auditory.
Cradle Plays				
Cradle Play*	Kiddicraft	C	Chain Stores, Dept Stores, Toy Shops, etc.	Eye and Hand co-ordination. Good value.
Play Gym	Fisher-Price	E	Only available in USA at present	Eye and Hand co-ordination. Attractive perspex centre. Robust.
Mirrors				
Play Mirror*	Kiddicraft	B	Chain Stores, Dept Stores, Toy Shops, etc.	Visual.
Baby Mirror*	Abbott (ESA)	B	ESA Catalogue	Visual.
Baby-see Mirror*	Mothercare	B	Mothercare Shops or Catalogue	Visual.
Fish Mirror*	—	B	Boots	Visual.
Pram Rattle Toy	Mothercare	B	Mothercare Shops or Catalogue	Reaching. On elastic. To be strung across pram.
Pram Beads	Kiddicraft	B	Chain Stores, Dept Stores, Toy Shops, etc.	Reaching. On elastic.
Pram People	Kiddicraft	B	Chain Stores, Dept Stores, Toy Shops, etc.	Reaching. Bell rattles on elastic.

Toy	Supplier or Manufacturer	Price	Availability	Comments
Rattles				
Ring a Ling teether	Pedigree	B	Chain Stores, Dept Stores, Toy Shops, etc.	Rattle and teether.
Happy Smile Rattle	Kiddicraft	B	Chain Stores, Dept Stores, Toy Shops, etc.	Rattle and teether with revolving ball in centre.
Dumbel Rattles*	Kiddicraft	B	Chain Stores, Dept Stores, Toy Shops, etc.	Two rattles in pack.
Bangle Rattle	Kiddicraft	B	Chain Stores, Dept Stores, Toy Shops, etc.	Teething ring with interesting attachments that slide round.
Fingers and Tongue Rattle*	Kiddicraft	B	Chain Stores, Dept Stores, Toy Shops, etc.	Very popular. Pleasant sound.
Swirl Rattle	Kiddicraft	B	Chain Stores, Dept Stores, Toy Shops, etc.	For two handed play.
Wobble Globe*	Kiddicraft	B	Chain Stores, Dept Stores, Toy Shops, etc.	Popular suction rattle.
Click a Wheel	Kiddicraft	B	Chain Stores, Dept Stores, Toy Shops, etc.	For encouraging two-handed play.
Flip Fingers*	Kiddicraft	B	Chain Stores, Dept Stores, Toy Shops, etc.	Encourages use of two hands.
Happy Rattle (Butterfly Rattle)	Playskool	B	Some Chain Stores, Dept Stores and Toy Shops	Transparent wings provide fascination.
Bird Rattle	Playskool	B	Some Chain Stores, Dept Stores and Toy Shops	Same principle as flip fingers but in shape of a bird. For two handed play.
Baby Mirror	Playskool	B	Some Chain Stores, Dept Stores and Toy Shops	Cross between a mirror and a rattle.
Ball in Circle	ESA	A	ESA Catalogue	Wooden ball in wooden circle. Pleasant feel.
Three Ball Rattle	—	A	Boots and other Shops	Very light. Nice sifting noise.
Dick Bruna Rattles	Corgi	B	Some Shops	Spinning centre with Dick Bruna character.

Toy	Supplier or Manufacturer	Price	Availability	Comments
Rumba Safety Rattle*	Mothercare	B	Mothercare Shops and Catalogue	Very popular design.
Rota Rattle	–	B	Hamleys Shop and Catalogue, various Shops	Suction rattle with three spinning arms that clatter as they go round.
Spinning Rattle	–	B	Hamleys Shop and Catalogue, various Shops	Suction rattle with four perspex balls that spin round.
Flower Rattle*	Fisher-Price	B	Chain Stores, Dept Stores, Toy Shops, etc.	Popular sturdy rattle cum teether with mirror, heavier than some rattles.
Baby Butterfly	Fisher-Price	B	Chain Stores, Dept Stores, Toy Shops, etc.	Attractive rotating parts.
Roll Rattle	Galt	A	Galt Catalogue and Shops	Wooden cage rattle with bell inside.
Bell Cube	Galt	A	Galt Catalogue and Shops	Wooden cube with bell inside.
Animal Squeakers	Galt	A	Galt Catalogue and	Coloured vinyl.
Grip hedgehog	–	A	Boots, ESA	Interesting texture, squeaks when squeezed.
Drill Bells*	Galt	A	Galt Catalogue and Shops	Bells on wooden rod.
Jingle Bells	Galt	B	Galt Catalogue and Shops	Bells on semi-circular strip with wooden handle.
Maracas*	Galt	B	Galt Catalogue and Shops	Bright red. Very light. Attractive sound.
Japanese Wooden Face Rattle	Japan	B	Toy and Craft and Novelty Shops	Lovely echoing sound. Wooden. Not for strong chewers!
Clic Clac Rattle*	Kiddicraft	B	Chain Stores, Dept Stores, Toy Shops, etc.	Excellent design. Tube with pieces that slide up and down. Nice clacking sound.
Whirly 3	Mothercare	B	Mothercare Shops and Catalogue	Three stem suction toy.

Dangling Toys

Toy	Supplier or Manufacturer	Price	Availability	Comments
Jumping Jack* Scarecrow	Fisher-Price	C	Chain Stores, Dept Stores, Toy Shops, etc.	Visual and Auditory. stimulation.

Toy	Supplier or Manufacturer	Price	Availability	Comments
Pull a Tune Bluebird	Fisher-Price	D	Chain Stores, Dept Stores, Toy Shops, etc.	Plays tune when handle is pulled.
Musical Rabbit	Kiddicraft	D	Chain Stores, Dept Stores, Toy Shops, etc.	Plays tune when handle is pulled.
Cot Toy	—	C	Hamleys Shops and Catalogue	Pooh pops out when string is pulled.
Chirpy Bird	Mothercare	B	Mothercare Shops and Catalogue	Bounces up and down on elastic cord and chirps.
Activity Centres				
Activity Centre*	Fisher-Price	D/E	Chain Stores, Dept Stores, Toy Shops etc.	Excellent toy that can be attached to cot. Several activities.
Turn and Learn Activity Centre	Fisher-Price	D	Chain Stores, Dept Stores, Toy Shops, etc.	Turns on revolving base. Several activities. Very sturdy.
Activity Box	Playskool	D	Some Shops	Stable base with several activities.
Roly-Polys				
Roly-Poly Chime	Mothercare	B	Mothercare Shops and Catalogue	Early reaching and pushing. Chimes.
Happy Apple	Fisher-Price	C?	Chain Stores, Dept Stores, Toy Shops, etc.	Early reaching and pushing. Chimes.
Chime Ball*	Fisher-Price	C	Chain Stores, Dept Stores, Toy Shops, etc.	Very popular and sturdy. Rings and chimes.
Balls				
Easy Grip Type	Various including Mothercare and ESA	B	Mothercare Shops and Catalogue; ESA Catalogue; other shops	Bright colours and ridges to grip. Often squeak.
Musical Ball	Various including ESA	B	Various Shops; ESA Catalogue	Easy to grip.
Flutterball*	Playskool and others	C	Various Shops	Not for rough use. Visually fascinating perspex ball with rotating inner butterfly.
Baby Action Ball*	Playskool	C	Various Shops; ESA Catalogue	Easy to grip. Visual and auditory interest.

Toy	Supplier or Manufacturer	Price	Availability	Comments
Discovery Ball	Four to Eight	C	Four to Eight Catalogue	Dismantles. Good clacking sound as it rolls. Not for rough use.
Perforated Plastic	Galt and other	A	Shops and Galt Catalogue (gamester ball)	Very light easy grip ball.
Soft Ball	Mothercare and various others	B	Mothercare Shops and Catalogue	Has ribbon for hanging in cots, etc. Tinkles when shaken.
Coloured Patchwork Balls (set of four)	ESA	C	ESA Catalogue	Bright colours, soft material. Bells inside.
Comeback Roller	Mothercare	B	Mothercare Shops and Catalogue	Rolls forward then back. Elastic bands may get broken by some children.

Pull-alongs

Toy	Supplier or Manufacturer	Price	Availability	Comments
Kouvalias Cricket, Mushrooms, Windmill*	Kouvalias	D	Various Shops	Excellent toy. Very sturdy and attractive. Good for children with poor co-ordination.
Drum Rattle	Brio	C	Various Shops and Tridias Catalogue	Wooden body with separate rotating cage rattle.
Bob-along Bear*	Fisher-Price	C/D	Chain Stores, Dept Stores, Toy Shops, etc.	Fascinating toy with twirling arms.

Others

Toy	Supplier or Manufacturer	Price	Availability	Comments
Tilting Tabby	Playskool	C	Various Shops	Cat with two handles. Eyes and mouse move as it is tilted.
Tambourine	Galt and others	C	Galt Catalogue; various Shops and Music Shops	Good for encouraging two handed play. Get a well made one like the Galt one with firmly attached bells.

FOR TODDLERS

Toy	Supplier or Manufacturer	Price	Availability	Comments
Early Fitting Tunnel Pegs	ESA	D	ESA Catalogue	Sturdy first fitting toy.
Pop up Toy*	Galt	C	Galt Catalogue and Shops	Fascinating first fitting and colour matching toy with bouncing peg men.
Clic'n Clatter Car	Fisher-Price	C?	Chain Stores, Dept Stores, Toy Shops, etc.	Lovely toy with revolving front wheel and telephone dial type back wheels. Large man ideal for fitting.

(All Escor toys wooden, well finished and brightly painted.)

Toy	Supplier or Manufacturer	Price	Availability	Comments
Baby Car (and various other cars)	Escor	B?	Escor Catalogue	Simple wooden car, bright colours. Man for fitting.
Rowing Boat	Escor	B?	Escor Catalogue	Sturdy base. Three men to fit.
Merry-Go-Round*	Escor	D?	Escor Catalogue	Four cars with driver on revolving platform. Ideal for fitting and later for language and imaginative play. Very popular.
Charabanc	Escor	D	Escor and Galt Catalogues	Eight men for fitting and imaginative play.
Roundabout*	Escor	D	Escor and ESA Catalogues	Two chairs and two horses with riders that can be spun round. Harder fitting as riders have to be fitted into pegs. Language and imaginative play.

Toy	Supplier or Manufacturer	Price	Availability	Comments
Graded Fitting and Stacking Nesting Beakers (Building beakers)*	Mothercare, Kiddicraft, Playskool and others	B	Various Shops; Mothercare Catalogue	Versatile and popular toy.
Stacking Rings	Pedigree	B	Various Shops	Popular.

Toy	Supplier or Manufacturer	Price	Availability	Comments
King of the Castle (Stacking Castles)	Pedigree	B	Various Shops	Notched tops make them better for stacking than ordinary beakers. King can be used for language games.
Rainbow Tree	Kiddicraft	B	Various Shops	Brightly coloured take apart tree with five size graded rings.
Stacking Clown	Kiddicraft	C	Various Shops	Rocking base, rings, body, head and hat stack on central rod.
Rock-a-Stack*	Fisher-Price	B/C	Chain Stores, Dept Stores, Toy Shops, etc.	Very simple stacking toy with brightly coloured size graded rings.
Clown	Brio	D	Galt and E.S. Arnold 'Offspring' Catalogues; Some Shops.	Brightly coloured wooden pieces.
Pyramid Rings	Merit	B	Various Shops	Good value basic graded stacking toy.
Posting Boxes Cube posting box	Galt	C	Galt Catalogue and Shops	Traditional wooden posting box with spare pieces.
Abbott Posting Box	ESA	B	ESA Catalogue	Good value basic wooden posting box.
Shape Sorter*	Fisher-Price	D	Chain Stores, Dept Stores, Toy Shops, etc.	Stable and sturdy plastic posting box with little doors to open.
Posting Box	Kiddicraft Mothercare and others	B	Chain Stores, Dept Stores, Toy Shops etc.	Good value basic plastic posting box.
Teddy Bear Post Box*	Playskool	C	Some Shops	Lovely plastic posting box in shape of a teddy bear with a hat for lid.
Posting Bucket	Orchard Toys	B?	Some Shops	Versatile posting toy as bucket can also be filled and emptied in the normal way and used to carry things around.
Shape O'Ball	Tupperware	C?	Tupperware Agents	Greater range of shapes for harder shape matching. Novel posting ball with pull apart handles.

Toy	Supplier or Manufacturer	Price	Availability	Comments
Royal Mail Post Van	Galt	D	Galt Catalogue and Shops	Wooden. Bright red. Can also be used as a push and pull along and therefore provides more interest than a traditional posting box.
Posting House	Susan Wynter	C	Susan Wynter Catalogue	Wide base and slide back pieces make it useful for poorly co-ordinated children.
Play Fit pull along truck	Mothercare	C	Mothercare Shops or Catalogue	Colourful plastic pull along posting toy provides extra interest.
Shape Register**	Palitoy	D?	Various Shops	Excellent toy. Provides interest to shape matching but should not be handled too roughly.

Early Colour Matching

Toy	Supplier or Manufacturer	Price	Availability	Comments
Pop up Toy*	Galt	C	Galt Catalogue and Shops	Interesting early colour matching and fitting toy.
Abacus Balls	Escor	D?	Escor Catalogue and ESA Catalogue	Bright coloured balls in five basic colours that fit onto rods.
Cash Register**	Fisher-Price	D	Chain Stores, Dept Stores, Toy Shops, etc.	Excellent toy. Makes colour matching exciting and interesting. Also teaches the child other activities such as turning the handle.
Climbing Clowns*	E.S. Arnold and others	B and C	E.S. Arnold, 'Offspring' Catalogue and some Shops	Versatile toy useful for colour matching, easy stacking and language play.

Early Construction and Building

Toy	Supplier or Manufacturer	Price	Availability	Comments
Lincabricks	Galt	E	Galt Catalogue and Shops	Giant size plastic bricks easy to fit together. Twenty-four in a set.

Toy	Supplier or Manufacturer	Price	Availability	Comments
Click-fit Bricks*	Tupperware	B?	Tupperware Agents	Square plastic bricks hinged so that they open. Can be joined to half of next brick and so on. In three basic colours so useful for colour discrimination, finding games and two handed play.
Building Bricks	ESA and others	B	ESA Catalogue and Shops	Brightly coloured wooden bricks.
First Building Bricks	ESA, Galt and others	C	ESA and Galt Catalogues	Brightly coloured cubes, slats and half cubes in wood for building early houses etc.
Truck of Bricks	Galt and others	C	Galt Catalogue	Twenty coloured wooden bricks in wooden pull along.
Floot-a-toota	Kiddicraft	C	Chain Stores, Dept Stores, Toy Shops, etc.	Twelve pieces that fit together to make a long plastic trumpet.

Early Joining, Threading and Screwing Toys

Toy	Supplier or Manufacturer	Price	Availability	Comments
Giant Snaplock Beads	Fisher-Price	B?	Chain Stores, Dept Stores, Toy Shops, etc.	Large brightly coloured plastic beads that snap together and pull apart. Good for two handed play.
Threading Beads*	ESA	B	ESA Catalogue	Beautiful translucent solid plastic beads with stiff thick plastic rope for easy threading. Also useful earlier for visual tracking.
Twist'n Turn	Kiddicraft	B	Chain Stores, Dept Stores, Toy Shops, etc.	Large easy to turn pieces make this a good starting toy.
Billie & his Barrels	Kiddicraft and others	B	Various Shops	Several plastic barrels that consist of two halves that screw together. Size graded with Billie in the middle. Good for teaching screwing and unscrewing.

Toy	Supplier or Manufacturer	Price	Availability	Comments
Screwing Rod	Galt	B	Galt Catalogue and Shops	Plastic rod with ten plastic nuts.

Surprise or Cause and Effect Toys

Toy	Supplier or Manufacturer	Price	Availability	Comments
Pop up Cone Tree* or Trigger Jigger*	Pedigree Mothercare	B	Various Shops Mothercare Catalogue and Shops	Excellent surprise toys with plastic cones that shoot off a plastic rod when the trigger is touched. Spring tends to get broken if treated inappropriately.
Pop up Humpty Dumpty	Pedigree	C	Various Shops	Same principle as pop up cane but this time six-part Humpty is shot in the air.
Pop up Rocket	Kiddicraft	C	Chain Stores, Dept Stores, Toy Shops, etc.	Four stage rocket with spaceman and nose cone which is fired from a base.
Surprise Box**	?	C or D?	Various Shops	Excellent toy for encouraging manipulation. Various devices such as a lever, a knob and a dial have to be operated to make sections with plastic animals inside fly open. Does not stand up to very rough play.
Jack in the Box**	Fisher-Price	C/D	Chain Stores, Dept Stores, Toy Shops, etc.	Very popular. Jack flies out of box when knob is pressed. Requires two hands to push him back and close lid.
Frisky Frog	Fisher-Price	C?	Chain Stores, Dept Stores, Toy Shops, etc.	Frog jumps when bulb is squeezed, good for language work. Tendency for tubing to break if treated roughly.
Farmer Giles*	Palitoy	D?	Various Shops	Fascinating and easy to use toy. Keys are pressed to make various animals pop out of their homes.

Toy	Supplier or Manufacturer	Price	Availability	Comments
Musical Toys				
Music Box Radio	Fisher-Price	C?	Chain Stores, Dept Stores, Toy Shops, etc.	Very robust and popular fascination toy, knob rather stiff. Choose from one of three tunes.
Two Tune Music Box TV	Fisher-Price	D	Chain Stores, Dept Stores, Toy Shops, etc.	Very robust. Good fascination toy but only encourages a limited type of play activity. Knob rather stiff.
Big Mouth Singers**	Palitoy	D/E	Various Shops	Excellent toy. Easy to use and attracts the attention of many children who are difficult to interest in toys.
Burbank Jack in the Box	Burbank	D?	Various Shops	Plays a tune when handles turned. Jack flies out of metal box at the end of the tune. Less suitable for destructive children.
Kermit Jack in the Box	—	D?	Various Shops	Plays a tune when handle is turned. Two tiers with small Kermit on top spring out at the end of the tune with a loud noise. May frighten some children but others love it. Not particularly robust.
Playslide**	Matchbox	E	Various Shops	Lovely toy. Good for manipulative and language play. When the handle is turned a tune plays and little people go up the moving steps and down the slide.
Musical Fire Engine*	Kiddicraft	D	Chain Stores, Dept Stores, Toy Shops,	A bright plastic versatile toy. Swivelling xylophone ladder, two bells and a drum skin mounted on push-along body.
Xylotruck	Mothercare	C	Mothercare Catalogue and Shops	Xylophone mounted on plastic truck.

Toy	Supplier or Manufacturer	Price	Availability	Comments
Pull a Tune Xylophone*	Fisher-Price	D	Chain Stores, Dept Stores, Toy Shops, etc.	Plays a tune when pulled along. Keys are colour coded so that older children can play tunes.
Music Box Record Player*	Fisher-Price	E?	Chain Stores, Dept Stores, Toy Shops etc.	Good toy for teaching a sequence of activities. Plays ten different tunes. No needle, touch plastic records and parts stand up well to energetic treatment.
Musical Ferris Wheel	Fisher-Price	D/E	Chain Stores, Dept Stores, Toy Shops, etc.	When wound up wheel with people in seats revolves as music plays. Good for language games.
Melody Train	Palitoy	D	Chain Stores, Dept Stores, Toy Shops, etc.	Plays a tune as it goes round the xylophone like tracks (these can be rearranged to play different tunes).
Carousel	Corgi		Chain Stores, Dept Stores, Toy Shops, etc.	Rotating musical roundabout with five removable figures. Attractive toy but somewhat limited play value.
Fascination Toys Novelty Tops	ESA	C	ESA Catalogue and some Shops	Lovely half perspex spinning tops with visible moving objects such as a train inside. Very attractive but fairly fragile.
Spinning Top (Kaleidoscope)	Mothercare	B	Mothercare Shops and Catalogue	Three individual discs on main top result in a kaleidoscope of colour when top is spun. Fairly fragile.
Traditional Metal Spinning Tops	–	B-C	Top Shops, Chain Stores and Dept Stores	Cheaper ones tend to break easily but good ones should be more robust.

Toys	Supplier or Manufacturer	Price	Availability	Comments
Bubble Blowers	—	A-B	Widely Available	Great fun. Look for special non-spill containers.
Kaleidoscope	ESA and others	A-B	ESA Catalogue and various Shops	Only suitable for children who can be persuaded to hold it up close to their eye.
Plastic Slinky	ESA	B	ESA Catalogue	Larger than metal slinky.
Builda-Helta Skelta*	Kiddicraft and ESA	C	ESA and Kiddicraft Catalogues, various Shops	Excellent toy. Good for social, co-operative and language games. Sometimes successful with children who generally show little interest in toys.
Flutterball*	Playskool	B	Toy Shops, Dept Stores, Chain Stores	Lovely toy, large perspex ball with rotating butterfly. Rather fragile.
Twurtle	Palitoy		Toy Shops, Dept Stores and Chain Stores	Friction toy turtle with colourful rotating back.
Pull- and Push-alongs				
Melody Push Chime	Fisher-Price	C	Toy Shops, Dept Stores and Chain Stores	Sturdy chiming push-along.
Rattle Ball	Fisher-Price	B	Toy Shops, Dept Stores and Chain Stores	Fascinating push-along to watch as beads rotate in clear plastic globe. Nice sound as well.
Little Snoopy (also Giant Snoopy)*	Fisher-Price	C	Toy Shops, Dept Stores and Chain Stores	All time favourite. Makes a loud clic clac noise as it goes along. Springy tail.
Chatter Telephone	Fisher-Price	C	Toy Shops, Dept Stores and Chain Stores	Makes a pleasant clacking sound as pulled along and eyes rotate. Can be used as an ordinary toy telephone as well.
Clatterpillar*	Kiddicraft	C	Toy Shops, Dept Stores and Chain Stores	Lovely toy. Bright coloured durable plastic. Fascinating movement and clattering sound.

Toy	Supplier or Manufacturer	Price	Availability	Comments
Energetic Play				
Rocking Boat	Galt ESA	E	ESA and Galt Catalogues	An ideal 'first-seesaw' as it is non-tip with bucket seats.
Nursery Trampoline	Galt ESA	E	Galt and ESA Catalogues and Shops	Special small trampoline with a hold on bar for younger children. Very popular.
Swing Safety Seat	Galt	C	Galt Catalogue	Wooden safety seat with ropes that can be attached to ordinary swing frame.
Plastic Hoops	Galt ESA	A-B	Galt and ESA Catalogues and Shops	Ideal for a variety of games.
Safety Baby Walker	ESA	E	ESA Catalogue	Specially designed non-tip baby walker.
Push & Ride Bear	Mothercare	D	Mothercare Catalogue and Shops	Nice colourful toy that can be used by one or two children to push or ride along.
Snuggle Egg	ESA	E	ESA Catalogue	Completely enclosed plastic seal makes this a useful toy for nervous or unsteady children.
Nursery Rocker	Galt	E	Galt Catalogue	Expensive but attractive wooden rocking horse with semi-enclosed seat.

(For babywalkers, sit and push-along and pedal type toys it is best to shop around as prices vary considerably. Second hand solid wooden baby walkers and rocking horses are worth considering as new ones tend to be expensive. Mothercare have an attractive range of plastic sit and push type toys. Many department and chain stores and mail order firms such as Argos also have a range of attractive plastic sit push type toys at reasonable prices. Always check that the toy is stable and robust and the right size for your child.)

Social, Imaginative and Imitative Play

Models				
Tea Set	ESA and others	B	ESA Catalogue and Shops	Useful for encouraging all these types of play.
Hoover	ESA	C	ESA Catalogue	Realistic model for encouraging imitation.
Carpet Sweeper	ESA	B	ESA Catalogue	Realistic model for encouraging imitation.

Toy	Supplier or Manufacturer	Price	Availability	Comments
Kitchen Set*	Galt	D	Galt Catalogue	Expensive but very attractive and robust set of aluminium pans. A favourite in our Toy Library.
Kitchen Set*	Fisher-Price		Dept Stores, Chain Stores and Toy Shops	Two ring cooker top and with dishes and utensils and a plastic tablecloth.
Telephone	Galt, E.S. Arnold, ESA and others	B	Relevant Catalogues and many Shops	Basic red plastic telephone with working dial and bell. A great favourite. Good for language and social play.
Merry-go-Round*	Escor	D	Escor Catalogue and Toy Shops	Beautiful painted wooden revolving roundabout with four detachable cars and men. A great favourite. Very versatile and robust. Not suitable for children who throw a lot without super-vision as cars are heavy!
Roundabout	Escor	E	Escor Catalogue and Toy Shops	Colourful revolving wooden roundabout with four people seated on two horses and two chairs. Both the Roundabout and the Merry-go-Round are excellent for language play.
Tree House**	Palitoy	E	Toy Shops, Dept Stores and Chain Stores	Versatile plastic dolls house with swing, lift, car, kennel and retract-able stairs. Ideal for language and imaginative play. Very popular toy but less suited to heavy-handed children.

Toy	Supplier or Manufacturer	Price	Availability	Comments
Playslide*	Matchbox	E	Various Shops	Also mentioned under musical toys. Good for language and social play. Younger children often need help to use this toy initially.
Weeble Playground		D	Various Shops	Good for language and imaginative play. Not very durable.
Joggle Train	Palitoy	E	Various Shops	Colour Train and passengers. Language and Imaginative play.
Family Ferry	Matchbox	C	Various Shops	Plastic boat with detachable figures. Fairly robust.
Family Camper	Matchbox	C	Various Shops	Plastic Truck, boat and trailer with detachable figures. Language and Imaginative play.
Play Family Fun Set	Fisher-Price	B	Various Shops	Good basic language and fitting toy. Very popular with children.
Play Family Airport	Fisher-Price	E	Various Shops	Good models with working parts.
Play Family Garage	Fisher-Price	E	Various Shops	Imaginative and language play.
Play Family House*	Fisher-Price	E	Various Shops	Good value plastic dolls house with furniture. Imaginative and language play.
Pictures, Lottos, etc.				
Talking Pictures	ESA	C	ESA Catalogue	Large plastic coated photographs on cards of everday objects. Very clear. Useful for early picture recognition and naming.
Giant Picture Lotto*	ESA	C	ESA Catalogue	Excellent first lotto with bright clear pictures. Social and language play.

Toy	Supplier or Manufacturer	Price	Availability	Comments
Giant Picture Snap	ESA	C	ESA Catalogue	Bright clear pictures are interesting and appealing. Makes a good early language toy before it is used for playing 'Snap'.
Books				
'Things I see' series, e.g. traffic, animals	Galt	A	Galt Catalogue and Shops	Clearly printed colourful pictures on very thick board that is hard to rip. Early language.
About the House Book	Philip & Tacey	A	Philip & Tacey Catalogue	Inexpensive but flimsy book. Clear pictures of a wide variety of household objects. Several to a page. Useful for word recognition, e.g. 'Where's the teapot?'
First Sentence Book Cards	LDA	C	LDA Catalogue	Cards make up eleven books of two word sentences round which the adult weaves a story. Amusing drawings.
Baby's First Book ABC Book Picture Book	Ladybird	A	Various Shops	Popular books. All have clear pictures of objects. For basic recognition and naming.
Talkabout series, e.g. The home, The garden, Shopping, etc.	Ladybird	A	Various Shops	Most topics relevant to a child's daily life. Useful for expanding language.
First Words Picture Book	Methuen	B	Bookshops	Covers the fifteen topics that young children talk about first and most often. Beautiful colour photographs.
First Picture 1 " " 2 Learn to Look 1 " " 2	Barnaby Books LDA	B	LDA Catalogue	Printed on heavy card. Suggestions and ideas for teaching with each book.
Look and See Books, e.g. Bedtime, Mealtime, My Clothes, Playtime*	Methuen	A	Various Shops	Very clear uncluttered photographs on card. All of familiar objects and activities in a young child's life.

Toy	Supplier or Manufacturer	Price	Availability	Comments
Miscellaneous				
Kermit Puppet	Several	B-D	Various Shops	Open and close mouth, long arms and legs, make it ideal for imitative and language play. Can be frightening to some children initially. Can be used for a whole variety of imitative language and social games.
Animal Clock	Mattel	D	Various Shops	Turn the arrow to select an animal picture pull the cord and hear the sound it makes. Useful for early imitation and naming.
Pocket Camera	Fisher-Price	C	Various Shops	Twenty-seven slides of a Trip to the Zoo ideal for picture recognition and naming.

Puzzles that are Useful for Encouraging Language

(Nearly all these simple jigsaws are mounted on wood and stand up well to wear and tear.)

Toy	Supplier or Manufacturer	Price	Availability	Comments
See Inside Jigsaws* Shops Cars Farm	Galt	C	Galt Catalogue and Shops	Excellent first inset with five or six lift out pieces such as cars and lorries on the traffic tray. Pieces have small knob for lifting out. Very popular with children.
Stand Up Jigsaws* Farm Zoo	Galt	C	Galt Catalogue and Shops	The Farm has 14 liftout animals on a clear background. Pieces are raised for easy lifting out and can be stood up. Ideal for early sound imitation and naming. A great favourite in our Toy Library.
Abbatt Inset Puzzles Garden House Kitchen Cupboards	ESA	C	ESA Catalogue and good Toy Shops	'See Inside' type insets. Lift out pieces such as the cupboard doors and see the picture inside. Pieces have knobs.
Picture Trays Country Traffic	ESA	D	ESA Catalogue	Large trays with several large clear lift out pieces.

Toy	Supplier or Manufacturer	Price	Availability	Comments
Meal Time Jigsaws Breakfast Lunch Tea Supper	Four to Eight	C	Four to Eight Catalogue	Clear photographic prints mounted on wood. Action in each picture. Useful for expanding understanding and putting words together.
Everyday Object Pictures Dustpan & Brush Telephone Teapot & Cups, etc.	Four to Eight	C	Four to Eight Catalogue	Photographic print puzzles with between two and 14 pieces. Very clear and attractive to children.
Inset Puzzles* Teatime Circus	Susan Wynter	B	Susan Wynter Catalogue and good Toy Shops	Lovely insets in 3D. Pieces can be taken out and stood up. Good for action words and prepositions as well as labelling.
Tray Jigsaws Clothes Pots'n Pans	Sysan Wynter	B	Susan Wynter Catalogue and good Toy Shops	Pieces all fit in a frame. Lots of pictures on each tray around one theme.
Raised Inset Puzzles* Breakfast Washing	John Adams Toys	B	John Adams Catalogue	Chunky easy to lift pieces are big enough for early imitative and imaginative play as well as encouraging language.
Transport Insets Bus Road Traffic Train	E.S. Arnold	C	E.S. Arnold Catalogue	See Inside type insets. Bright clear pictures are more complicated than any of the previous puzzles. Useful for expanding parts of speech.
Colour Picture Puzzles*	ESA	C	ESA Catalogue	A set of big simple two piece interlocking puzzles. Colour matching one side and picture matching the other side.
Giant Floor Jigsaws Autumn Forest, etc.	ESA	B	ESA Catalogue	Fifteen piece colourful interlocking jigsaws printed on wood. Fairly complicated pictures.
Floor Jigsaw Fruit Vegetables	Galt	C	Galt Catalogue and Shops	Fifteen piece wooden jigsaws. Nice clear pictures of fruit and vegetables with uncluttered background.
Giant Jigsaws Jungle Woodland	Galt	C	Galt Catalogue and Shops	Fifteen piece clear but fairly complicated pictures.

NURSERY AND INFANT

Toy	Supplier or Manufacturer	Price	Availability	Comments
Colour and Shape Matching				
Posting Pagoda*	Kiddicraft	C	Various Shops	Popular toy with colour matching keys, doors, roofs and shapes.
Balloon Lotto	Dick Bruna	B	Some Shops	Simple colour matching game with colour dice.
Hickory Dickory Dock*	Orchard Toys	B?	Some Shops	Delightful colour matching game with colourful cardboard clocks and mice.
Early Birds	Kiddicraft	B	Various Shops	Simple colour matching game with colour dice.
Mr Postman	Palitoy	D	Various Shops	Lovely toy with sorting machine and post van that delivers coloured letters to matching coloured houses.
Keys of Learning	Palitoy	C	Various Shops	Coloured keys unlock coloured blocks when correctly matched.
Ladybird, Ladybird*	Orchard Toys	B	Various Shops	Excellent game. Fun way of learning basic counting.
Insey Winsey Spider	Orchard Toys	B	Various Shops	Popular simple game involving counting.
What Time is it Mr Wolf	Orchard Toys	B	Various Shops	Simple game that children love to play.
Racing Home*	Kiddicraft	B	Various Shops	Slightly more complicated but involves much rehearsal of numbers one to four.
One Dozen Eggs	Palitoy		Various Shops	Match eggs by numbers.
Number and Sets Lotto	Galt	B	Galt Catalogue and Shops	Practise of numbers one to five.
Count and Match Lotto	Galt	B	Galt Catalogue and Shops	Practise of numbers one to five.
Count to 20	Galt	B	Galt Catalogue and Shops	Practise at counting up to 20.
Number Me*	Galt	B	Galt Catalogue	Enjoyable game involving numbers 1-10.

Toy	Supplier or Manufacturer	Price	Availability	Comments
Fit-a block Clock	Mothercare	C	Mothercare Shops and Catalogue	Clear removable figures for learning numbers.
Puzzle Numerals	ESA	B	ESA Catalogue	Match number to dots 1-10.
Colour Matching Dominoes	Galt	B	Galt Catalogue and Shops	Clear wooden dominoes with colours to help to match numbers.
Cash Register	Galt	D	Galt Catalogue and Shops	Imaginative and social games involving numbers.

Constructional Toys

Toy	Supplier or Manufacturer	Price	Availability	Comments
Sticklebricks (various size sets)	Galt, ESA and Playskool	C-D-E	Catalogues and Shops	Bricks mesh together and wheels can be added. Fairly easy to use.
Octons*	Galt	B	Galt Catalogue and Shops	Attractive translucent coloured plastic pieces that slot together to form abstract shapes.
Nursery Octons	Galt	C	Galt Catalogue and Shops	Polythene pieces are more durable but less attractive than translucent octons.
Constructo-Straw	ESA	B	ESA Catalogue	Requires fine co-ordination to make attractive abstract constructions.
Take apart Work Bench or Big Tool Bench	Playskool	E	Some Shops	Expensive but well made with lots of play value.
Jigbits	Kiddicraft	B	Various Shops	Attractive cardboard pieces slot together to make circus figures, wild animals, etc.

Games

Toy	Supplier or Manufacturer	Price	Availability	Comments
Scardey Cat*	Orchard Toys	B	Various Shops	Exciting game. Collect as many birds as possible before the cat scares them away (4-10 years).
Cat & Mouse	Orchard Toys	B	Various Shops	Thought provoking game.

Toy	Supplier or Manufacturer	Price	Availability	Comments
Tummy Ache*	Kiddicraft	B	Various Shops	Great fun involving shape recognition and matching.
Jumble Sale*	Kiddicraft	B	Various Shops	Gives practise in shaping, matching and counting.
Giant Picture Dominoes	ESA	B	ESA Catalogue	Clear pictures on wooden dominoes to match up.
Alphabet Lotto	ESA	B	ESA Catalogue	Fun way of learning sounds.
Picture Lotto	Galt	B	Galt Catalogue and Shops	Enjoyable way to improve picture recognition and matching.
Lotto	Dick Bruna	C	E.J. Arnold Catalogue and some Shops	Enjoyable way to improve picture recognition and matching.

(All LDA packs have suggestions on how to use the material.)

Language

Toy	Supplier or Manufacturer	Price	Availability	Comments
Action Cards Sets 1, 2 & 3*	LDA	B	LDA Catalogue	Simple pictures designed to encourage action words and short sentences.
Photographic Action Cards	LDA	B	LDA Catalogue	Simple photographs encourage action words.
Prepositions	LDA	B	LDA Catalogue	Photographs to encourage use of prepositions and verbs (e.g. he's *climbing over* the wall).
Spatial Relationship Concept Cards	LDA	B	LDA Catalogue	Useful for teaching in, on, under, behind, in front, etc.
Help Yourself Books 1-4 e.g. Girl Dressing	LDA	B	LDA Catalogue	Suggestions with each page to develop language and understanding of everyday activities.
Picture Word Lotto	Galt	B	Galt Catalogue and Shops	Picture matching and word matching.
Say What You See Cards	Galt	B	Galt Catalogue and Shops	Pictures to describe and compare in spot the difference game.

Toy	Supplier Manufacturer	Price	Availability	Comments
Chameleon Street	Philip & Tacey	E	Philip & Tacey Catalogue	Whole set of pieces including human figures, cars, etc. that can be arranged to make pictures that can be talked about.
Drawing and Writing				
Play desk	Fisher-Price	D/E	Various Shops	Small desk with handle, chalk, magnetic letter and numbers and stencils. Fun way to encourage early drawing and writing.
Magnetic Figures	Galt and other	C	Galt Catalogue and various Shops	Use colourful wooden pieces with built in magnets to make pictures.
Plywood Templates Transport Home and Garden Domestic Animals etc.	Galt	B	Galt Catalogue	Wooden shapes to draw round.
Templates Animals Transport etc.	Orchard Toys	B	Various Shops	Simple cardboard templates to draw round.
Imaginative				
Magnetic Theatre	ESA and others	C	ESA Catalogue and some Shops	Delightful theatre with two sets of scenery and figures that are moved around the stage by means of magnetic rods.
Glove Puppets	ESA and others	B	ESA Catalogue and various Shops	Lovely puppets that promote imaginative and language play.
Playmats Roadway Dale Farm	ESA and Galt	E	ESA and Galt Catalogues and various Shops	Attractive mats with clearly marked roads, houses, etc. on a large scale. Hardwearing. Lots of play value.
Motor Master	E.J. Arnold and Matchbox	C	E.J. Arnold Catalogue and Shops	Cardboard pieces that slot together to form a roadway.
Hob	E.J. Arnold	D	E.J. Arnold Catalogue	Large hob with four rings and switches.

Toy	Supplier or Manufacturer	Price	Availability	Comments
Play Family Village	Fisher-Price	E	Various Shops	Two streets with 32 pieces including a fire station, a post office and post van, a theatre and a garage with car lift. Lots of scope for imaginative play.
Lift & Load Depot	Fisher-Price	E	Various Shops	Working model that will fascinate children who like mechanical toys.
Rescue Centre	Palitoy	E	Various Shops	Lots of activity when the buttons are pressed.
Wild Animals	Four to Eight	C	Four to Eight Catalogue	Two hundred layout, fences and animals.
Play People Sets Builders Doctors & Nurses Cowboys Firemen Farm etc.	Galt and others	C (per set)	Galt Catalogue and various Shops	Model people with moveable limbs can be manipulated to carry out a variety of activities. For children who enjoy complex imaginative play and will not treat the pieces too roughly.

Thinking and Cognitive

Toy	Supplier or Manufacturer	Price	Availability	Comments
Picture Clues	LDA	C	LDA Catalogue	Enjoyable way of trying to guess what an object is when only part of it can be seen. Flaps are opened in turn to reveal gradually more of it. Ideal for social and language games as well.
Things that go together	LDA	B	LDA Catalogue	Match pictures of needle and thread, hammer and nail, etc.
What's wrong cards	LDA	B	LDA Catalogue	Pictures of silly things like a bicycle with square wheels. Encourages thinking and language.
Sequential Thinking	LDA	B	LDA Catalogue	Put the cards in order to tell a simple story like making tea.

Toy	Supplier or Manufacturer	Price	Availability	Comments
Classification of Objects	LDA	B	LDA Catalogue	Encourages concept of categories such as, building, flowers, etc. that pictures can be divided into.
Find it	Galt	B	Galt Catalogue and Shops	Match card by association to the correct board, e.g. cooking utensils in the kitchen and wash things in the bathroom. Encourages abstract thinking and can be played as a game.
Pair it	Galt	B	Galt Catalogue and Shops	Match card to base board by association, e.g. bat to ball, key to lock, etc.

(See also the games section. These are an excellent way of encouraging thinking and concept formation and can often be used successfully with children who find these more formal activities boring.)

SPECIAL NEEDS

PHYSICALLY HANDICAPPED CHILDREN

Toy	Supplier or Manufacturer	Price	Availability	Comments
Babies				
Kouvalias Toys* e.g. Windmill Cricket Mushroom	Kouvalias	C-D	Various Shops	Lovely toys. Very attractive with bright coloured balls that wobble and clatter on strong springs when swiped at. Ideal for children with poor hand and arm control.
Flutterball	Playskool	B	Various Shops	Attractive light clear perspex ball with butterfly inside. Will roll easily. Useful for following with eyes and practising swiping. Fairly fragile.

Toy	Supplier or Manufacturer	Price	Availability	Comments
Turn and Learn Activity Centre	Fisher-Price	D	Various Shops	Revolves on base. Can be set in motion with a swipe.
Activity Centre*	Fisher-Price	D/E	Various Shops	Can be screwed to a cot or other furniture so it stays in place when a child is attempting to do various activities on it.
Activity Box	Playskool	D	Various Shops	Wide base and easy to revolve rod on to top.
Cradle Play*	Kiddicraft	C	Various Shops	Pieces revolve easily. Ideal for encouraging grasping and swiping.
Pram People	Kiddicraft	B	Various Shops	Colourful and easy to swipe at.
3-Ball Rattle	—	A?	Boots and other Shops	Very light rattle, thin plastic frame between balls can be easily grasped.
Come back Roller	Mothercare	B	Mothercare Catalogue and Shops	Very light and easy to set in motion with a swipe.
Whirly 3	Mothercare	B	Mothercare Catalogue and Shops	Useful as suction base stops it being knocked out of child's reach. Can be tried with children who dislike holding rattles.
Wobble Globe*	Kiddicraft	B	Various Shops	Popular Suction Rattle that is easy to set in motion and makes an attractive sound.
Chime Ball	Fisher-Price	C	Various Shops	For encouraging kicking whilst lying down as well as swiping. A bit heavy for some children but has the advantage of not often rolling out of reach.
Pull a Tune Bluebird	Fisher-Price	C	Various Shops	Large handle fairly easy to pull. Will probably need help initially. Should encourage more accurage reaching and grasping.

Toy	Supplier or Manufacturer	Price	Availability	Comments
Jumping Jack*	Fisher-Price	C	Various Shops	(Comments as above.) Very attractive to watch as well.
Musical Rabbit	Kiddicraft	D	Various Shops	(Comments as above.)
One and Over				
Morgenstern Arched Abacus*	ESA	D	ESA Catalogue	Sturdy wire hoop with colourful wooden balls and wooden base. Very robust. Popular with many children because balls cannot get 'lost'.
Pop up Men*	Galt	C	Galt Catalogue and Shops	Very popular toy. Wooden men bounce up and down in their slots if hit. For reaching and grasping.
Tunnel Pegs*	ESA	C	ESA Catalogue	Sturdy and versatile first fitting toy. Pegs rather large for some hands.
Abacus Balls	Escor	D	Escor Catalogue and good Toy Shops	Colourful shiny wooden balls on rods. For encouraging reaching, grasping and releasing.

Musical Toys

(See under previous musical toy headings. Especially recommended tambourines, maracas and drill bells.)

Toy	Supplier or Manufacturer	Price	Availability	Comments
Big Mouth Singers**	Palitoy	D	Various Shops	Excellent toy. Switch on and use fist or fingers to press keys and open singers' mouths. Quite often successful with children who rarely play with toys.
Giant Picture Snap*	ESA	C	ESA Catalogue	Bright clear pictures for encouraging finger or eye pointing.
Magic Music Maker	Kiddicraft		Various Shops	Press large keys to play tunes.

Toy	Supplier or Manufacturer	Price	Availability	Comments
Leybourne Mirror Frame	Four to Eight	C	Four to Eight Catalogue	Large tough mirror with two easy grip handles particularly suitable for handicapped children.
Leybourne Colour Frame	Four to Eight	C	Four to Eight Catalogue	Three different colour frames each with two easy grip handles.
Rock a Stack	Fisher-Price	B	Various Shops	Colourful plastic rings on central cone. For encouraging accurate hand and arm movements.
Farmer Giles	Palitoy	D	Various Shops	Delightful press button toy that can be operated with index finger or fist.
Rescue Centre	Palitoy	D/E	Various Shops	Everything works at the push of a button. For encouraging use of finger.
Playdesk	Fisher-Price		Various Shops	Magnetic letters can be arranged on magnetic desk.
Magnetic Figures	Galt	C	Galt Catalogue and various Shops	Colourful wooden pieces can be used to make a picture on the magnetic board. Will probably need help at first.
Picture Printing*	Galt	C	Galt Catalogue and Shops	Very popular with most children and can be very rewarding for brighter physically handicapped children.
Pastry Cutters	Galt	A	Galt Catalogue	Very popular with most children and can be very rewarding for brighter physically handicapped children.
Sticklebricks (Various size sets)	Galt, ESA and others	C-D-E	Catalogues and Shops	Bricks mesh together at any angle so easier to use than many conventional stacking bricks.

Toy	Supplier or Manufacturer	Price	Availability	Comments

Puzzles and Insets

(Look under previous headings for these and choose ones with knobs or raised pieces.)

Toy	Supplier or Manufacturer	Price	Availability	Comments
Giant Knob Puzzles 3 ladybirds 3 cats etc.	Globe Education	C/D	Globe Education; some Shops	Wooden puzzles made in Belgium with extra large knobs.
Stayput Jigsaws Sets 1-4	Philip & Tacey	C (set of 6)	Philip & Tacey Catalogue	Magnetic puzzles with between 20 to 42 pieces. Pieces fit onto tray and are held in place by magnetic force so they are less likely to be accidently knocked.

Special Toys

Toy	Supplier or Manufacturer	Price	Availability	Comments
With adapted switches fitted to a variety of conventional battery operated toys which move, light up and make noises when switched on.	Toy Aids	D/E	Toy Aids	A special switch is fitted consisting of a large flat square of wood which makes contact with slight pressure. Ideal for any child with poor hand and arm control.
including:				
Patrol Plane		E		
Flying Saucer		E		Lights up and moves in circles.
Fighting Robot		E		Sparks and Flashes as he moves.
Fire Chief Car		E		Liked by many children.
Telemax TV		E		A variety of film strips can be used with it.
Melody Train		E		Plays tune as it goes round the track. Popular. Good for stop/go games.

Two-handed Play

Toy	Supplier or Manufacturer	Price	Availability	Comments
Click a Wheel	Kiddicraft	B	Various Shops	Have to hold in two hands in order to rotate wheels and produce clicking.
Flip Fingers	Kiddcraft	B	Various Shops	Hold in one hand, flip moving parts with other hand.

Toy	Supplier or Manufacturer	Price	Availability	Comments
Bird Rattle	Playskool	A	Various Shops	Hold in one hand, flip moving parts with other hand.
Tilting Tabby	Playskool	B	Various Shops	Hold in two hands and tilt in order to see Tabby watching moving mouse.
Threading Beads*	ESA	B	ESA Catalogue	Attractive translucent beads and thick plastic thread.
Billie and his Barrels*	Kiddicraft and others	B	Various Shops	Favourite screw and unscrew toy.
Twist 'n' Turn	Kiddicraft	B	Various Shops	For screwing and unscrewing.
Flootatoota	Kiddicraft	C	Various Shops	Fit pieces together.
Jack-in-the-Box	Fisher-Price	D	Various Shops	Need two hands to get Jack back in the box.
Radio	Fisher-Price	D	Various Shops	Turn stiffish knob.
Two Tune Music Box TV	Fisher-Price	D	Various Shops	Turn stiffish knob to hear tune and see moving picture. Limited in scope but very popular with some children.
Pocket Camera	Fisher-Price	C	Various Shops	Excellent toy for involving use of two hands in children who enjoy looking at pictures.
Triola	Galt	C	Galt Catalogue and Shops	Hold in one hand and blow using other to press keys.
Constructional Toys e.g. Jet Plane Roundabout Swingboats Construction Set	Escor	D-E	Escor Catalogue and good Toy Shops	Lovely wooden toys. Construction set is particularly versatile making into a lorry. fire engine or charabanc. Pieces fixed together with plastic nuts.
Constructs-Straw	ESA	B	ESA Catalogue	Fine co-ordination between both hands required.
Mr Climb	Susan Wynter	A	Susan Wynter Catalogue	Excellent and inexpensive toy for encouraging two-handed play. Buy two and have races at getting Mr Climb to the top.

Toy	Supplier or Manufacturer	Price	Availability	Comments
Easy Grip Scissors	ESA	C	ESA Catalogue	Easy to hold scissors which require the minimum of pressure to work.

DEAF CHILDREN

Most of the toys listed under language, imaginative and social play.

Also listed musical toys. Ask you peripetetic teacher of the deaf for advice on musical toys and other noise producing toys to ensure that you use those that are at an appropriate sound level for your child.

The Toy Libraries Association produce an excellent booklet called 'Hear and Say' with advice on toys and activities for children with hearing, speech and language difficulties.

VISUALLY HANDICAPPED CHILDREN

Toy	Supplier or Manufacturer	Price	Availability	Comments

BLIND

(Most noise producing rattles — see listing under Babies.)

Toy	Supplier or Manufacturer	Price	Availability	Comments
Wobble Globe*	Kiddicraft	B	Various Shops	Popular suction rattle with attractive sound.
Chime Ball	Fisher-Price	C	Various Shops	Makes a nice sound and does not roll far out of reach.
Action Ball	Playskool	C	Various Shops	Soft sifting sound, interesting shape. Does not roll far.
Musical Ball	ESA	B	ESA Catalogue	Easy to grip.
Discovery Ball	Four to Eight	B	Four to Eight Catalogue and some Shops	Come apart ball makes a sound as it rolls along and has a removable rattle.
Activity Centre**	Fisher-Price	D/E	Various Shops	Many noise producing activities on it. Can be fixed in place.
Pull a Tune Bluebird	Fisher-Price	D	Various Shops	Big handle to grip and pull.
Musical Rabbit	Kiddicraft	D	Various Shops	Pull handle to play tune.

Toys	Supplier or Manufacturer	Price	Availability	Comments
(Musical Toys: Most of those previously listed such as tambourines, drums and bells and wind up and battery operated toys like the Big Mouth Singers and the Fisher-Price radio.)				
Hedgehog	—	A	Various Shops	Plastic hedgehog with soft spines and a squeak.
Feely Bags	—		Home-made	Make in a variety of textures and fill with a variety of dried materials such as peas, rice, pearl barley.
Feely Box	—		Home-made	Fill a cardboard box with a variety of crumpled paper, tissue paper, corrugated paper, balls of wool, cotton reels; anything in fact that has an interesting texture or makes an interesting sound.
Chirpy Bird	Mothercare	C	Mothercare Shops and Catalogue	Soft furry bird with felt feet and beak and shiny eyes to feel. Chirps as he bounces up and down on elastic cord.
Soft Ball	Mothercare and others	B	Mothercare Shops and Catalogue and other Shops.	Soft textured ball with chime.
Coloured Patchwork Balls (Set of 4)	ESA	C	ESA Catalogue.	Various shape and size soft balls with built in bells.
Feely boards and Scraps	—		Home-made	As many different texture materials and surfaces either pasted onto individual pieces of board or on their own (e.g. velvet, foil, polystyrene, sandpaper, cord, etc.).
Nursery Trampoline*	ESA and Galt	E	ESA and Galt Catalogues	Special holding handle makes these safe for blind children to use. Ideal way of encouraging movement and burning up energy.

Toy	Supplier or Manufacturer	Price	Availability	Comments
Hoover	ESA	C	ESA Catalogue	Large model hoover that whirs as it goes along. Interesting to explore with hands.
Morgenstern Arched Abacus	ESA	D	ESA Catalogue	Balls on hoop cannot get lost and make an interesting thud as they reach the base.

OLDER BLIND CHILDREN

Toy	Supplier or Manufacturer	Price	Availability	Comments
Play house Cleaning Set	ESA	D	ESA Catalogue	Different texture brooms and brushes, mop and a sponge and a carpet sweeper make this an interesting set to explore.
Hammer Balls	Galt	C	Galt Catalogue and Shops	Interesting toy with balls disappearing through holes and reappearing. Helps to teach concept of going in and coming out.
Builda Helta Skelta	Kiddicraft	—	Various Shops	Marbles clatter down plastic runways.
Tactile Patterns	ESA	B	ESA Catalogue	Match plastic textures.
Touch a Shape	ESA	B	ESA Catalogue	Plastic shapes can be matched into board by texture.
Touch Tuner	Four to Eight	E	Four to Eight Catalogue	Match textures to board. Rather expensive version of the home-made feeling lotto.
Dunwell Frame*	ESA	C	ESA Catalogue	Special surface leaves a series of raised dots when a child draws on it so he can feel what he has drawn.
Pairing Bridges (4 Sets)	Philip & Tacey	C	Philip & Tacey Catalogue	Match bridges by textures or raised shapes.

PARTIALLY SIGHTED

Toy	Supplier or Manufacturer	Price	Availability	Comments
Flower Rattle	Fisher-Price	B	Various Shops	Brightly coloured.
Happy Rattle	Playskool	B	Some Shops	Fascinating translucent wings.

Toy	Supplier or Manufacturer	Price	Availability	Comments
Activity Centre	Playskool	D	Some Shops	Firm base, bright revolvable striped rod on top.
Cricket) Windmill) etc.)	Kouvalias	D	Various Shops	Bright glossy moving balls on springs will encourage looking and reaching.
Rock a Stack	Fisher-Price	C	Various Shops	Brightly coloured rings are easy to see.
Musical Roly Poly	Mothercare	B	Mothercare Shops and Catalogue	Brightly coloured.
Threading Beads	ESA	B	ESA Catalogue	Large bright beads and thread.
Plastic Dominoes	ESA	C	ESA Catalogue	Large white dominoes with black spots.
Sand and Water Play Bath Harbour	Kiddicraft	B	Various Shops	Popular bath toy with simple suction harbour and boats.
Bathtime Fun Centre	Berwick?	D	Various Shops	Like an activity centre but with water involved in all the activities. Not very robust.
Sand pit	E.J. Arnold	D	E.J. Arnold Catalogue	Attractive tough plastic sandpit that doubles up as a paddling pool.
Sand Tray	E.J. Arnold	D	E.J. Arnold Catalogue	For floor play or cover to the sand pit. Has moulded hills, roads, etc.
Toy Sieve	ESA	A	ESA Catalogue	Plastic sieve.
Water Syphon	ESA	B	ESA Catalogue	Real pump.
Sand and Water Wheel*	ESA and Galt	B	ESA and Galt Catalogues and various Shops	Great fun. Can also be used with dried lentils on a tin tray or box. Makes a nice noise.
Sand Play Set	ESA	C	ESA and Galt Catalogues and various Shops	Nice set with moulds, sieve spades, water-wheel and buckets.
Stacking Castles	Galt and others	B	Galt Catalogue and various Shops	Five plastic sand-castles can be used for stacking as well.

Toy	Supplier or Manufacturer	Price	Availability	Comments
Playscoops*	Galt and others	B	Galt Catalogue and various Shops	Popular set of nesting plastic pans with handles.
Bathducks*	Kiddicraft	B	Various Shops	Three floating plastic ducks that join together and serve as scoops.

Play Development Charts

	Activity	Toys
6 weeks	Begins social play with mother of looking 'stilling' and movement.	
10-12 weeks	Hand–eye co-ordination first seen in finger play.	Mobiles
14 weeks	Can hold and look steadily at a small toy given to him.	
18-20 weeks	Can reach and grasp an offered rattle using whole palm.	Rattles
	Can shake rattle, take it to mouth and withdraw it.	
	Can drop rattle by opening hands but not place it down.	
	Can hold rattle between two hands.	
6 months	Stretches to grasp a toy.	Cradle plays.
7 months	Can hold a small toy or object in both hand simultaneously.	Roly-Poly's Chime Ball
	Can pass a toy from hand to hand.	
	Starts to look for a toy hidden in front of him.	
	Will drop a plaything and watch with interest to see how and where it falls.	
	Bangs and slides toys on surfaces to produce sounds.	
9-10 months	Stretches out an arm to grasp a dangling toy or pick up an object from floor.	Activity Centres
	Pokes toy or object with index finger.	Pull-a-tune, Bluebird and other pull cord toys
	Grasps small toys and objects between thumb and finger in a scissor like manner.	
	Can take wooden pegs out of holes.	Galt Pop-up Toy, ESA Tunnel Pegs and other simple fitting toys
10-12 months	Starts to use pincer grip (i.e. to pick up small objects with thumb and index finger).	Nesting beakers Simple posting boxes and stacking toys

	Activity	Toys
10-12 months (cont)	May start to show a hand preference (i.e. to be right or left handed).	Pull-alongs
	Enjoys sound making toys and performs appropriate activity to reproduce the sound.	
	Pushes and pulls large toys.	
	Will imitate activities such as ringing a bell or rattling a spoon in a cup.	
	Imitates adult 'play type' vocalisations with enjoyment.	
	Gives a toy to an adult when asked and sometimes spontaneously.	
	Plays social games such as pat-a-cake.	
	Starts to show an interest in pictures.	Giant Snap Cards and books with clear pictures
	Exploratory play begins in earnest.	
15 months	Uses pincer grasp well to pick up small objects.	Pop-up cone
	Holds a crayon and imitates scribble.	Simple insets and jigsaws
	Builds a tower of two cubes.	
	Enjoys putting objects in and out of containers.	Big size cars, engines and trucks
	Short episodes of role play with dolls' house, teaset, etc.	Large dolls and largish models of household objects such as a teaset
18 months	Enjoys simple picture book (turns several pages at a time).	
	Enjoys nursery rhymes and tries to join in.	Telephone
	Several single words uses appropriately and some phrases such as 'gimme' (give me).	
	Can point to parts of his or adult's body such as nose, hair, eyes, etc.	
	Obeys simple instructions.	Musical toys
	No longer takes toys to mouth.	
	Very interested in examining small objects and looking into boxes, drawers, bags, etc.	
2 years	Can use push- and pull-along toys competently.	Simple model toys with a few people, e.g. Fisher-Price aeroplane or Escor roundabout
	Can build a tower of six or seven cubes.	
	Spontaneous circular scribble. Can imitate a vertical line.	
	Recognises fine detail in picture books, names and turns pages singly.	Picture books
	Usually definitely right of left handed by now.	Crayons
		Sand and water play toys

	Activity	Toys
2 years (cont)	Can ride a small push-along with feet type toy and steer it.	Large size construction toys such as Giant Lego or Climbing Clowns
	Puts two or more words together to form a simple sentence.	
	Constantly asks names of people and objects.	
	Experiments for long periods of time with materials like water, sand, clay, but not able to plan or produce an end product.	
	More pretend play.	
	Understands what miniature toys (e.g. dolls' house size or model car size) represent and how to play with them.	
3 years	Can match three or more primary colours.	Jigsaws, insets; more complicated colour matching toys such as Fisher-Price Cash Register
	Can match several shapes.	
	Can copy a circle and draw a very primitive man with a head.	Simple lottos, picture and colour dominoes
	Can cut with scissors.	
	Enjoys a wide variety of 'educational' toys such as formboards, posting boxes, fitting toys.	All sorts of fitting toys, e.g. Fisher-Price Play Family Toys
	Enjoys listening to stories.	Simpler model garages, dolls' houses, etc., e.g. Palitoy Tree House
	Can repeat several nursery rhymes.	
	More prolonged and elaborate make-believe play.	
4 years	Able to count out about five objects accurately.	Dolls' houses, Farm Sets, Garages and the like
	More elaborate drawing of a man usually having head, body, legs, arms and/or features.	Weeble sets
	Shows increasing skill at ball games.	Pedal Bike
	Very adventurous and may well climb ladders and trees.	Giant Floor Jigsaws
	Can pedal a bike easily.	Fisher-Price Playdesk
	Constructive building with large material.	Sticklebricks, Octons, Lego
	Enjoys a variety of constructional toys.	Construct-a straw
	Can do more complicated jigsaw puzzles.	Colouring books, modelling clay, paints, etc.
	Plays well with miniature toys such as dolls' house or farm set.	
	Enjoys early 'rule' games such as snap and picture lotto.	Picture Lotto, Scaredy Cat Insey, Winsey Spider, etc.
	Plays with other children and co-operates in games like shops, cars, hospitals, schools etc.	

Addresses to Write to for Advice and Information

1. Associations for Handicapped Children and Their Parents

Association for All Speech-impaired Children (AFASIC),
Toynbee Hall, 28 Commercial Street, London E1 6LS.
(Tel: 01-247 1497)

Association for Research into Restricted Growth,
2 Mount Court, 81 Central Hill, London SE19 1BS.

Association for Spina Bifida and Hydrocephalus,
Tavistock House North, Tavistock Square, London WC1 9HJ.

Association of Parents of Vaccine-damaged Children,
2 Church Street, Shipston-on-Stour, Warwicks CV36 4AP.

Association to Combat Huntingdon's Chorea,
6 Widecombe Court, Lyttleton Road, London N2.

British Diabetic Association,
3-6 Alfred Place, London WC1E 7EE.
(Tel: 01-636 7355)

British Council for the Rehabilitation of the Disabled,
Tavistock House (South), Tavistock Square, London WC1H 9LB.
(Tel: 01-387 4037)

British Dyslexia Association,
18 The Circus, Bath, Avon BA1 2E7.

British Epilepsy Association,
3-6 Alfred Place, London WC1E 7EE.
(Tel: 01-580 2704)

British Sports Association for the Disabled,
Stoke Mandeville Stadium, Harvey Road, Wylesbury, Bucks HP21 8PP.
(Tel: 0296 84848)

British Institute for the Achievement of Human Potential,
Lanrick House, Wolseley Road, Rugeley, Staffs WS15 2QT.
(Tel: Rugeley 6511)

Brittle Bone Society,
63 Byron Crescent, Dundee DD3 65.

Central Council for the Disabled,
34 Eccleston Square, London SW1V 1PE.
(Tel: 01-837 0747)

Chest and Heart Association,
Tavistock House, Tavistock Square, London WC1H 9LB.

Cystic Fibrosis Research Trust,
5 Blyth Road, Bromley, Kent BR1 3RS.
(Tel: 01-461 7211)

DES (Dept of Education and Science) Publications,
Government Buildings, Honeypot Lane, Stanmore, Middlesex.

DHSS (Dept of Health and Social Security) Publications,
Government Buildings, Honeypot Lane, Stanmore, Middlesex.

Disabled Living Foundation,
346 Kensington High Street, London W14 8NS.
(Tel: 01-602 2491)

Family Fund,
Beverley House, Shipton Road, York YO3 6RB.
(Tel: 0904 29241)

Friedreichs Ataxia Group,
Bolsover House, 5/6 Clipstone Street, London W1.
(Tel: 01-636 2042)

Haemophilia Society,
PO Box 9, 16 Trinity Street, London SE1.
(Tel: 01-407 1010)

Handicapped Adventure Playground Association,
3 Oakley Street, London SW3.
(Tel: 01-352 2321)

Invalid Children's Aid Association,
126 Buckingham Palace Road, London SW1W 9SB.
(Tel: 01-730 9891)

Lady Hoare Trust for Physically Disabled Children,
7 North Street, Midhurst, W. Sussex GU29 9DJ.
(Tel: 073-081 3696)

Leukaemia Society,
28 Eastern Road, London N2.
(Tel: 01-883 4703)

Multiple Sclerosis Society,
4 Tachbrook Street, London SW1V 1SJ.
(Tel: 01-834 8231)

Muscular Dystrophy Group of Great Britain,
Nattrass House, 35 Macaulay Road, London SW4 OQP.
(Tel: 01-720 8055)

National Association for Deaf/Blind and Rubella Handicapped,
164 Cromwell Lane, Coventry CV4 8AP.
(Tel: 0203 462579)

National Deaf Children's Society,
31 Gloucester Place, London W1.
(Tel: 01-486 3251)

National Society for Autistic Children,
1A Golders Green Road, London W1.
(Tel: 01-453 4375)

National Society for Mentally Handicapped Children,
Pembridge Hall, 17 Pembridge Square, London W2 4EO.
(Tel: 01-229 8941)

Royal National Institute for the Blind,
224 Great Portland Street, London W1.
(Tel: 01-387 5251)

National Association for the Education of the Partially Sighted,
Joseph Clark School, Vincent Road, Highhams Park, London E4.
(Tel: 01-527 8818)

National Association for the Welfare of Children in Hospital,
7 Exton Street, London SE1.
(Tel: 01-261 1738)

2. Information Sources

National Bureau for Handicapped Students,
City of London Polytechnic, Calcutta House Precinct, Old Castle Street, London E1 7NT.
(Tel: 01-283 1030)

National Children's Bureau,
8 Wakley Street, London EC1 7QE.
(Tel: 01-278 9441)

National Eczema Society,
27 Doyle Gardens, London NW10 3DB.

National Physically Handicapped and Able-bodied,
42 Devonshire Street, London W1N 2AP.
(Tel: 01-580 4053)

Association for Special Education,
Beaconwood, Bordon Hill, Stratford-upon-Avon.

British Red Cross Society,
9 Grosvenor Crescent, London SW1.
(Tel: 01-235 5454)

Council for Children's Welfare,
183/189 Finchley Road, London NW3.
(Tel: 01-624 8766)

Dept of Health and Social Security (Information Division),
Alexander Fleming House, Elephant and Castle, London SE1.
(Tel: 01-407 5522)

Friends of the Centre for Spastic Children,
63 Cheyne Walk, London SW3 5NA.
(Tel: 01-352 8434)

Information Service,
Mary Marlborough Lodge, Nuffield Orthopaedic Centre, Headington, Oxford.

National Association for Mental Health,
22 Harley Street, London W1N 2ED.
(Tel: 01-637 0741)

National Children's Bureau,
1 Fitzroy Square, London W1P 5AH.
(Tel: 01-387 4263)

National College of Teachers of the Deaf, Secretary: Mr E. Brown,
Needwood School, Rangemore Hall, Burton-upon-Trent.

Royal National Institute for the Deaf Library,
105 Gower Street, London WC1.
(Tel: 01-387 8033)

Spastics Society Information Service,
16 Fitzroy Square, London W1P 5HQ.
(Tel: 01-387 9571)

National Society of Phenylketonuria and Allied Disorders,
6 Rawdon Close, Palace Fields, Runcorn, Cheshire.
(Tel: 092-85 65081)

Pre-School Playgroups Association,
Alford House, Aveline Street, London SE11 5DJ.
(Tel: 01-582 8871)

Scottish Information Service for the Disabled,
Claremont House, 18/19 Claremont Crescent, Edinburgh EH7 4QD.
(Tel: 031-556 3882)

Scottish Society for the Mentally Handicapped,
69 West Regent Street, Glasgow G2.
(Tel: 041-331 1551)

Spastics Society,
12 Park Crescent, London W1N 4EA.
(Tel: 01-636 5020)

Toy Libraries Association,
Seabrook House, Wyllyotts Manor, Darkes Lane, Potters Bar, Herts EN6 2HL.
(Tel: 0707 44571)

Down's Babies Centre (for mongol babies),
The Community Centre, Ridgacre Road, Quinton, Birmingham B32 2TW.
(Tel: 021-427 1374)

Gingerbread (for single parent families),
9 Poland Street, London W1.

Invalid Children's Aid Association
(all handicaps with a special interest in language disorders),
126 Buckingham Palace Road, London SW1.
(Tel: 01-730 9891)

National Association for Gifted Children,
27 John Adam Street, London WC2.
(Tel: 01-930 7731)

National Fund for Research into Crippling Diseases,
Vincent House, 1a Springfield Road, Horsham, Sussex.
(Tel: 0403 64101)

National Association for the Welfare of Children in Hospital,
7 Exton Street, London SE1.
(Tel: 01-261 1738)

Nursery School Association,
89 Stamford Street, London SE1.
(Tel: 01-928 7454)

Patients' Association,
335 Grays Inn Road, London WC1.
(Tel: 01-837 7241)

Riding for the Disabled Association,
c/o British Horse Society, National Equestrian Centre, Stoneleigh, Kenilworth, Warwicks.

Save the Children Fund,
29 Queen Anne's Gate, London SW1.
(Tel: 01-930 2461)

3. General

Advisory Centre for Education,
58 Russel Street, Cambridge.
(Tel: 51456)

Association of Occupational Therapists,
251 Brompton Road, London SW3.
(Tel: 01-589 7458)

Breakthrough Trust (for deaf and hearing),
19 Beaconsfield Road, New Malden, Surrey.

British Toy Manufacturers Association Ltd,
Regent House, 89 Kingsway, London WC2.
(Tel: 01-242 9158)

Chartered Society of Physiotherapy,
14 Bedford Road, London WC1.
(Tel: 01-242 1941)

College of Speech Therapists,
Harold Poster House, 6 Lechmere Road, London NW2 5BU.

List of Designers, Manufacturers and Suppliers

Paul and Marjorie Abbatt Ltd, 74 Wigmore Street, London W1. Catalogue now from: PO Box 22, Harlow, Essex CM19 5AY.

John Adams Toys Ltd, Crazies Hill, Wargrave, Berks. (Tel: Wargrave 3480).

E.J. Arnold & Son Ltd, Butterley Street, Leeds LS10 1AX.

Community Playthings, Robertsbridge, Sussex TN32 5DR (Tel: Robertsbridge 626).

Early Learning Centre, Hawksworth, Swindon SN2TT (Tel: 0793 431251).

Educational Supply Association, School Materials Division, Pinnacles, Harlow, Essex (ask for *Play Specials* and *Vital Years*) (Tel: Harlow 21131).

Escor Toys Ltd, Groveley Road, Christchurch, Hants. BH23 3RQ.

Fisher-Price Toys (Europe) Ltd, Lodge Farm Industrial Estate, Hopping Hill, Northampton NN5 7AW.

Four to Eight, Medway House, St Mary's Mills, Evelyn Drive, Leicester LE3 2BT.

Globe Education, Hounds Mills, Basingstoke, Hampshire RG21 2XS.

Denys Fisher Toys Ltd, Thorp Arch Trading Estate, Wetherby, Yorks. LS23 7BL (Tel: Boston Spa 843776).

James Galt & Co. Ltd, Brookfield Road, Cheadle, Cheshire SK8 2PN (Tel: 01-428 8511) (ask for Early Stages).

Goodwood Toys Ltd, Lavant, Chichester, Sussex (Tel: 0533-825626).

Hamleys, Regent Street, London W1.

Heal's, 196 Tottenham Court Road, London W1A 1BJ.

Huntercraft, ESA, PO Box 22, Harlow, Essex CN19 5AY (Tel: Harlow 21131).

Kiddicraft Ltd, Kenley, Surrey CR2 5YS (Tel: 01-668 1311).

Kooga, 12 St Lawrence Lane, Ashburton, Devon.

British Lego Ltd, Wrexham, Denbighshire.

Learning Development Aids, Park Works, Norwich Road, Wisbech, Cambs. PE13 2AX (Tel: Wisbech 2011).

London Music Shop, 218 Great Portland Street, London W1.

Merit Toys, J. & L. Randall Ltd, Cranborne Road, Potters Bar, Herts.

Mettoy Playcraft Co. Ltd, 14 Harleston Road, Northampton NN5 7AE.

Mothercare, Cherry Road, Watford, Herts. (for catalogue) and local branches.

Palitoy Ltd, Coalville, Leicester LE6 2DE (Tel: Coalville 3388) (ask for *Discovery Time* and the Parker catalogue).

Pedigree Toys, Market Way, Canterbury, Kent CT2 7JH.

Philip & Tacey Ltd, North Way, Andover, Hants. (showroom at 58 Fulham High Street, London SW6). (Will accept special orders from groups and organisations only — unless a special plea is made.)

Playforms, Relyon, Hospitals Division, Wellington, Somerset (Tel: Wellington 2216).

Playskool, Milton Bradley Ltd, CP House, 97-107, Uxbridge Road, Ealing, London W5 5TL (Tel: 01-567 3030).

Raleigh Toys, Raleigh Industries Ltd, Lenton Boulevard, Nottingham.

Tonka Ltd, 176 Park Avenue, London NW10.

Toy Aids, Lodbourne Farmhouse, Gillingham, Dorset.

Tridias, 8 Saville Row, Bath BA1 2QP, and at 44 Monmouth Street, London WC2.

Tupperware Co., 43 Grosvenor Street, London W1 (will provide local address list).

Woodpecker Toys, Burvill Street, Lynton, N. Devon (Tel: Lynton 2375).

Susan Wynter, Toy Trumpet Workshop, Brightlingsea, Essex.

(This list does not include firms which have branches thoughout the country. We suggest that you make a habit of dropping in to your local Boots, W.H. Smith, British Home Stores, etc. to see the current range of toys.)

Book List

Practical Guides

Cunningham, C. and Sloper, P. (1978) *Helping Your Handicapped Baby* (Souvenir Press)
Jeffree, Dorothy and McConkey, Roy (1976) *Let Me Speak* (Souvenir Press)
Jeffree, D., McConkey, R. and Hewson, S. (1977) *Let Me Play* (Souvenir Press)
Kiernan, C., Jordan, R. and Saunders, C. (1978) *Starting Off* (Souvenir Press)
(These four books are all written specifically for parents of handicapped children.)

Carr, Janet (1979) *I'm Handicapped — Teach Me* (Penguin)
Finnie, M. (1974) *Handling the Young Cerebral Palsied Child at Home* (Heinemann)
Gillham, Bill (1979) *The First Words Language Programme* (Allen & Unwin)
Lear, Roma (1977) *Play Helps: Toys and Activities for Handicapped Children* (Heinemann)
Newson, Elizabeth and Hipgrave, Tony (1982) *Getting Through to Your Handicapped Child* (Cambridge University Press)
Stone, J. and Taylor, F. (1977) *A Handbook for Parents with a Handicapped Child* (Arrow Books).
The Toy Libraries Association (1981) *The Good Toy Guide* (The Association also produces a number of useful pamphlets on various aspects of handicap and ways of helping through play.)

The National Society for Mentally Handicapped Children produce a number of useful leaflets plus a booklist on publications in mental handicap: see useful addresses.

Informative Books

General

Bowley, A. and Gardner, L. (1972) *The Handicapped Child* (3rd edition) (Churchill-Livingstone)
Hannam, C. (1975) *Parents and Mentally Handicapped Children* (Penguin Books)
Newson, John and Elizabeth (1980) *Toys and Playthings* (Penguin Books)
Sheridan, M, (1973) *Children's Developmental Progress* (NFER)
——— (1977) *Spontaneous Play in Early Childhood* (NFER)
Younghusband, E. *et al.* (eds) (1970) *Living with Handicap* (National Children's Bureau)

Visual and Hearing Handicaps

Fraiberg, Selma (1977) *Insights from the Blind* (Souvenir Press)
Freeman, Peggy (1970) *Understanding the Deaf/Blind Child* (Heinemann)
Gregory, Susan (1976) *The Deaf Child and his Family* (Allen & Unwin)

RNIB Pamphlet (n.d.) *Children with a Serious Visual Defect* (See useful addresses)
Tooze, Doris (1981) *Independence Training for Visually Handicapped Children* (Croom Helm)

Down's Syndrome

Carr, Janet (1975) *Young Children with Down's Syndrome* (IRMMH Monograph 4) (Butterworth)
Wilks, J. and E. (1973) *Bernard – Bringing Up Our Mongol Son* (Routledge & Kegan Paul)

Cerebral Palsy

Blencowe, S. (ed.) (1969) *Cerebral Palsy and the Young Child)* (Livingstone)
Hewett, S. (1970) *The Family and the Handicapped Child* (Allen & Unwin)

Autism

Wing, Lorna (1976) *Early Childhoon Autism* (Pergamon Press)

Aphasia

Browning, E. (1972) *I Can't See What You're Saying* (E. & K. Books Ltd)

Spina Bifida

Anderson, E. and Spain, B. (1977) *The Child With Spina Bifida* (Methuen)

About the Author

Barbara Riddick is a Senior Lecturer in the Department of Education, Trent Polytechnic. A qualified educational psychologist, she formerly ran the Nottingham University Toy Library and the Melrose Centre for Handicapped Children. Prior to working in the Child Development Research Unit at Nottingham University, she was Research Officer at the Thomas Coram Research Unit at London University where she was involved in researching and developing teaching programmes for the parents, teachers and nurses of handicapped children.

Index